Gastroesophageal Reflux Disease

A Clinician's Guide

First Edition

Gary Gitnick, MD, FACG
Professor of Medicine
Chief, Division of Digestive Diseases
UCLA School of Medicine
Los Angeles, California

Professional Communications, Inc. A Publishing Corporation

Published by:
Professional Communications, Inc.

For orders only, please call:
1-800-337-9838

ISBN: 1-884735-05-3

Library of Congress Card Number: 95-070371

Printed in the United States of America

This text is printed on recycled paper.

DEDICATION

This book is dedicated to those who have made it possible for me to devote time and effort to the development of books. They include my wife, Cherna; my children, Neil, Kim, Jill and Tracy; my brother, Jerry; and my mother, Ann.

ACKNOWLEDGEMENT

This book was made possible because of the efficient and dedicated work of Susan Dashe, the editorial coordinator in the Division of Digestive Diseases at UCLA; Jean Fitzpatrick, for her assistance in the preparation of the manuscript; Phyllis Jones Freeny, who coordinated the effort for Professional Communications, Inc.; Nikki D. Stewart, for her graphic design work; and Malcolm Beasley, whose inspiration and administrative skills made it all possible.

TABBED TABLE OF CONTENTS

TABLES

FIGURES

PART 1

INTRODUCTION TO GASTROESOPHAGEAL REFLUX DISEASE

Introduction

Gastroesophageal reflux, retrograde movement of gastric contents into the lower esophagus, is a transient, usually postprandial event that occurs undetected and without symptoms several times a day in healthy individuals.[1,2] How these benign incursions evolve into gastroesophageal reflux disease (GERD) was, until recently, believed to be related to the presence of a hiatal hernia and, like other so-called acid-peptic disorders, to too much gastric acid.[3,4] Now we know the mechanism is more complex, having to do primarily with the failure of the lower esophageal sphincter (LES) as an antireflux barrier. Furthermore, the essential cause of both symptoms and esophageal damage in GERD, unlike the other acid peptic disorders, is the displacement rather than the hypersecretion of acid.[3]

Gastroesophageal reflux disease, which accounts for 75% of esophageal pathology,[5] is characterized by a broad spectrum of clinical presentations, from simple heartburn to ulcerative esophagitis, esophageal stricture, and Barrett's metaplasia with its tendency to become malignant. Cross-sectional surveys of the adult US population have found that 7% to 10% have heartburn daily and 15% to 40% have heartburn monthly. Approximately one-third of the patients with heartburn who seek medical care have endoscopic evidence of esophagitis and about 10% to 20% have severe complications of esophagitis.[6]

The progression from transient reflux to heartburn to esophageal injury is dependent on a number of anatomic and physiologic factors associated with the structural and functional integrity of the LES.[7] This progression, as well as recent trends in epidemiology, pathogenesis, and management, are the subject of this text.

REFERENCES

1. Duke GE. Symposium: introduction. *Am J Hosp Pharm.* 1993;50(suppl 1):S3.

2. Ippoliti A. Inflammatory and infectious esophageal disorders. In: Gitnick G, ed. *Principles and Practice of Gastroenterology and Hepatology*, 2nd ed. Norwalk, Conn: Appleton & Lange; 1994:37-49.

3. Quigley EMM. Gastroesophageal reflux disease: the roles of motility in pathophysiology and therapy. *Am J Gastroenterol.* 1993;88:1649-1651. Editorial.

4. Rothstein RD. The ups and downs of gastroesophageal reflux disease. *Hosp Prac.* July 15, 1992:38-40.

5. DeMeester TR, Stein HJ. Gastroesophageal reflux disease. In: Moody FG, Carey LC, Jones RS, et al, eds. *Surgical Treatment of Digestive Disease.* Chicago, Ill: Year Book Medical Publishers; 1989:65-108.

6. Richter JE. Surgery for reflux disease—reflections of a gastroenterologist. *N Engl J Med.* 1992;326:825-827. Editorial.

7. Johnson DA. Medical therapy for gastroesophageal reflux disease. *Am J Med.* 1992;92(suppl 5A):88S-97S.

1 Natural History

1

Many patients with even severe reflux esophagitis may be symptomatic for months or even years before they seek medical help.[1] In one large series of 200 patients with severe disease, 18% had experienced significant symptoms for less than 1 year and 50% had been symptomatic for less than 3 years, but 24% had endured for more than 10 years.[2]

The frequency of spontaneous remission in gastroesophageal reflux disease (GERD) remains unclear, however.[3] Symptoms of the disease can improve, even disappear, without treatment.[4] Furthermore, GERD symptoms may differ in intensity over time, not correlated with the severity of esophagitis.

Studies that look at pharmacologic reduction of gastric acid have demonstrated that the majority of patients with reflux esophagitis remain in remission as long as therapy is continued.[5] In most patients, however, both symptoms and esophagitis return after treatment is stopped.

Despite its prevalence, chronicity, and propensity for complications, GERD rarely causes death.[2] In the study of 200 patients with severe esophagitis, for example, those followed for up to 16 years had the same mortality rate as that expected for a similarly aged group in the general population.[2]

REFERENCES

1. Wienbeck M, Barnert J. Epidemiology of reflux disease and reflux esophagitis. *Scand J Gastroenterol.* 1989;156 (suppl):7-13.

2. Brunnen PL, Karmody AM, Needham CD. Severe peptic oesophagitis. *Gut.* 1969;10:831-837.

3. Sontag SJ. Rolling review: gastro-oesophageal reflux disease. *Aliment Pharmacol Ther.* 1993;7:293-312.

4. Palmer ED. The hiatus hernia-esophagitis-esophageal stricture complex. Twenty-year prospective study. *Am J Med.* 1968;44:566-579.

5. Sontag S. The medical management of reflux esophagitis. Role of antacids and acid inhibition. *Gastroenterol Clin North Am.* 1990;19:683-712.

2

Pathophysiology

Healthy individuals experience, on the average, one to four episodes of gastroesophageal reflux per hour during the first 3 hours after a meal.[1] This normal physiologic reflux occurs as the lower esophageal sphincter (LES) relaxes in response to swallowing, occuring spontaneously at other times, and lasts up to 30 seconds.

The development and severity of gastroesophageal reflux disease (GERD) is contingent on the presence of three conditions:[1]

- Increased frequency of reflux
- Increased duration of reflux
- Injurious effects of gastric contents on the esophageal mucosa.

These conditions are created, in turn, by a process in which a variety of factors increase esophageal exposure to injurious gastric contents. One or more of several abnormalities may predominate in a given patient:[2]

- Compromised integrity of LES
- Increased nocturnal reflux
- Impaired esophageal clearance
- Increased intra-abdominal pressure
- Increased intragastric volume, acidity
- Gastric distention
- Duodenal-gastric reflux
- Gastric hypersecretion
- Injury to the esophageal tissue barrier
- Hiatal hernia.

Of these many contributory factors, the first, a structurally or functionally compromised LES is responsible in some degree for the development of the others. The majority of reflux episodes occur during so-called transient relaxations of the LES.[3] With increasing severity of esophagitis, however, absent basal LES pressure becomes a progressively more common mechanism, accounting for 23% of reflux episodes in patients with severe GERD.

The Role of the Lower Esophageal Sphincter

The LES is a unique band of smooth muscle fibers 2.5 cm to 4.0 cm in length, located partly in the abdomen and partly in the hiatal canal formed by the right crus of the diaphragm (Figure 2.1).[4] The LES, crural diaphragm, and phrenoesophageal ligament, which anchors the distal esophagus to the diaphragm, are the anatomic structures that comprise the gastroesophageal junction (GEJ), the anatomic barrier to reflux of gastric contents.

The LES normally maintains a resting pressure that is more than 12 mm Hg higher than the intragastric pressure, thus providing a barrier against the reflux of gastric contents.[5] It relaxes with the peristaltic wave initiated by a pharyngeal swallow before returning to its resting level.[6] Gastric juice that flows back through the open valve is rapidly cleared back into the stomach by a series of peristaltic contractions (Figure 2.2).[1,6]

Although gastroesophageal reflux may occur by any of several different mechanisms, the common denominator seems to be low sphincter tone, accounted for by either persistently low LES resting pressure or a transient LES relaxation.[7]

FIGURE 2.1—GASTROESOPHAGEAL JUNCTION

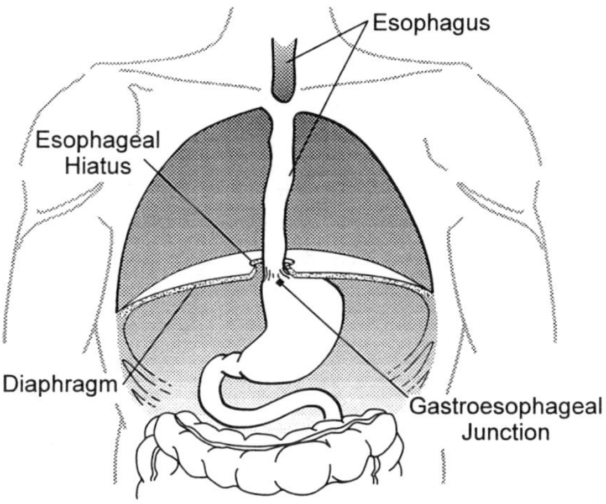

The lower esophageal sphincter, crural diaphragm, and phrenoesophageal ligament are the anatomic structures that comprise the gastroesophageal junction.

2

Transient Lower Esophageal Sphincter Relaxations

Transient LES relaxations (TLESRs), which may be spontaneous and not associated with any detectable motor activity, may follow immediately on either a normal peristaltic sequence or synchronous contraction in the esophageal body.[8] These apparently normal physiologic events are usually of longer duration than those associated with normal peristaltic waves and appear to be unrelated to basal LES tone. Only about 35% of TLESRs were associated with reflux in

FIGURE 2.2—ESOPHAGEAL MOTOR EVENTS DURING ACID REFLUX

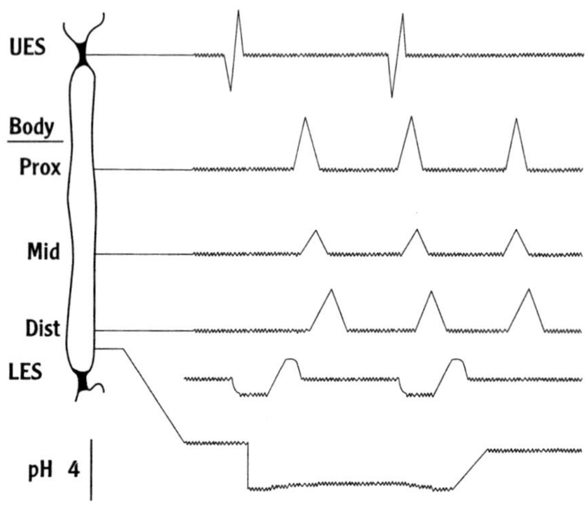

During relaxation of the LES, which was initiated by swallowing, acid reflux has occurred as indicated by the fall in esophageal body pH from the normal of between 6 and 7 to pH 4 or less. A series of peristaltic esophageal body contractions follow, the acid is cleared from the esophagus, and the pH returns to normal.

Ippoliti A. Inflammatory and infectious esophageal disorders. In: Gitnick G, ed. *Principles and Practice of Gastroenterology and Hepatology*, 2nd ed. Norwalk, Conn: Appleton & Lange; 1994:37-49. Reprinted with permission.

asymptomatic volunteers as compared to 65% in patients with GERD.

The factors that determine the occurrence of reflux during TLESRs are not completely understood.[8] However, their abrupt onset and brief duration suggest that they are neurally mediated. Studies in healthy volunteers have established that TLESRs are a normal response to gastric distention, the probable mechanism underlying the increase in both TLESRs and reflux episodes after meals.[8] Although the neural pathways involved have yet to be defined, current evidence favors a vagovagal reflex initiated by stimulation of mechanoreceptors in the gastric wall.

■ Mechanical Failure of the Lower Esophageal Sphincter

2

Mechanical dysfunction of the LES may be the result of abnormal pressure or, in a sphincter with normal pressure, of its inadequate length or position.

Inadequate LES pressure, the most common reason for mechanical failure, is probably caused by defective myogenic function.[6] The sphincter's intrinsic tone is modulated by neural and hormonal mechanisms. Esophagus and sphincter are innervated by both excitatory and inhibitory fibers from the vagus nerve, which seems to coordinate sphincter relaxation with esophageal contraction. Sphincter pressure is increased by some hormones, peptides, and pharmacologic agents, including antacids, and decreased by others, such as anticholinergics and theophylline. Peppermint, chocolate, coffee, ethanol, and fat are associated with reduced LES pressure, which may explain esophageal symptoms after a rich meal.[6]

Although a linear correlation between LES resting pressure and reflux has not been found, patients with severe disease often have extremely low LES resting pressures (< 5 mm Hg).[5]

■ Lower Esophageal Sphincter Length

A sphincter with normal pressure may also be compromised by either inadequate abdominal length or abnormally short overall resting length.[6] If the abdominal portion of the LES is too short, it may be unable to maintain resting tone during the increases in intra-abdominal pressure that occur with daily activities or changes in body position. When the overall resting length is inadequate, increases in gastric pressure caused by increased gastric volume or outlet obstruction may overwhelm the sphincter and cause reflux. Persons with such short sphincters are also vulnerable to postprandial reflux since normal dilatation of the stomach secondary to eating further shortens the already compromised LES.

Nocturnal Reflux

Although nocturnal reflux has been considered a significant factor in the pathogenesis of GERD, 24-hour pH studies have shown that the majority of patients with either mild erosive esophagitis or no endoscopic abnormality experience most reflux during the daytime postprandial periods.[9] The progressively greater acid exposure associated with more severe esophagitis is predominantly due to an increase in nocturnal reflux. The longest period of unbuffered basal gastric output occurs at night. This is due to both impaired clearance of acid from the esophagus and reduced neutralization by salivary bicarbonate. Sleep reduces both salivation and esophageal motility.[7,9,10]

Esophageal Clearance

Effective clearance of refluxed gastric contents from the esophagus is a two-step process.[11] Most of the refluxed gastric juice that gains entry through physiologic TLESRs is cleared from the esophagus by a primary peristaltic wave initiated by a pharyngeal swallow. The small amount of residual acid is neutralized by the bicarbonate in swallowed saliva.

Inadequate or delayed clearance, which results in prolonged esophageal exposure to gastric juice, is influenced by four major factors:[6,11]

- Defective esophageal motor activity
- Reduced salivation
- Absence of gravity's positive effects
- Loss of distal esophagus' intra-abdominal anchorage (hiatal hernia).[6]

■ Defective Esophageal Motor Activity

An estimated 48% of GERD patients with symptomatic esophagitis have esophageal peristaltic dysfunction.[12,13] A long-standing question has been whether this dysmotility precedes or is the result of reflux.[14] Although there is no definitive answer, evidence indicates that acid perfusion can induce a variety of esophageal motor abnormalities.[15,16] In a recent large study, for example, Crozier and colleagues found that in 90 of 275 patients (33%) with noncardiac chest pain and normal baseline manometry, their chest pain could be reproduced along with motor abnormalities (increased amplitude, increased duration, and simultaneous or spontaneous contractions) by acid perfusion.[16]

On the other hand, a number of studies have found no evidence that healing of esophagitis improves defective LES or esophageal body function, suggesting that the motor abnormalities precede the inflammation,[14] or that the change is irreversible.

■ Reduced Salivation

Depression of salivation provides less buffer to neutralize the microdroplets of acid that remain in the esophagus after a normal peristaltic contraction.[5] Salivary gland output may be compromised by:

- Smoking[12]
- Radiotherapy[6]
- Anticholinergic medications[12]
- Age[5]
- Sjögren's syndrome.

2

A drop in esophageal pH consequent to the reduction of salivary flow may initiate secondary peristaltic waves.[6] However, ambulatory motility studies indicate that these secondary waves have little effect on esophageal clearance. Their abnormal patterns actually reduce the efficiency of clearance and encourage regurgitation of refluxed material into the pharynx, predisposing the patient to aspiration.

Saliva production may increase in response to acid in the lower esophagus, resulting in hypersalivation, or "water brash," in some patients with severe reflux (Figure 2.3).[6,17]

■ Effect of Gravity

During sleep, without gravity's benefit, clearance is delayed.[11] Normal physiologic reflux may be further compromised by peristaltic dysfunction or reduced salivary flow.

■ Loss of Intra-Abdominal Anchorage

The close anatomical relationship of the structures that comprise the GEJ suggests an active role for the diaphragm in LES pressure and, in turn, prevention of reflux.

Some play in the intact phrenoesophageal ligament allows the distal esophagus to slide in and out of the diaphragmatic hiatus during esophageal peristalsis and LES relaxation.[4] In the presence of a hiatal hernia that does not reduce between swallows, however, esophageal clearance may be impaired during dynamic stresses such as swallowing and abrupt increases in abdominal pressure (see *Hiatal Hernia*, this section).[18]

Other Etiologic Factors

■ Intra-Abdominal Pressure

Stress-induced reflux occurs when intra-abdominal pressure overwhelms LES resting tone.[2] Squatting,

FIGURE 2.3—EFFECT OF PERFUSING THE ESOPHAGUS WITH N HCl IN PATIENTS WITH REFLUX ESOPHAGITIS

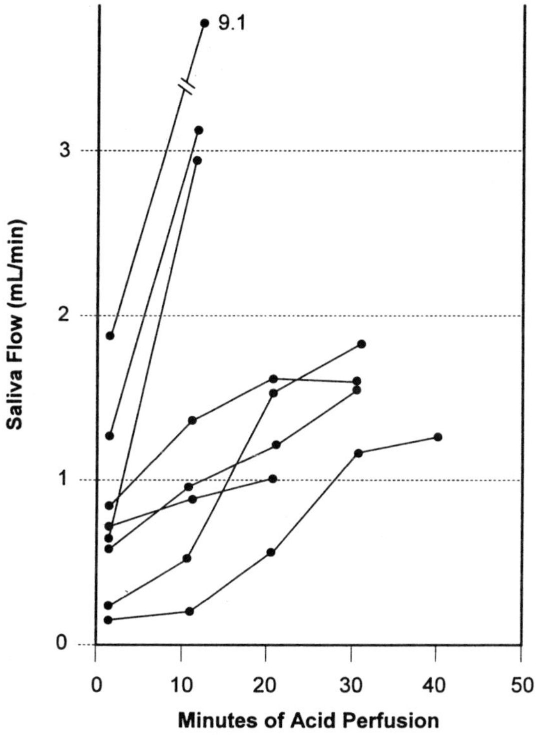

In patients with GERD, saliva flow increased concurrently with the onset of heartburn in response to infusion of the esophagus with 0.1 N HCl.

Helm JF, Dodds WJ, Hogan WJ. Salivary response to esophageal acid in normal subjects and patients with reflux esophagitis. *Gastroenterol.* 1987;93:1393-1397. Reprinted with permission.

2

stooping, and straining maneuvers are among the relatively common activities associated with transient physiologic reflux in healthy persons.[2,12] In patients with GERD, these common reflux triggers may exacerbate symptoms.

■ Gastric Volume

Increased gastric volume caused by overeating or slow gastric emptying may overcome the LES resting tone to increase the occurrence of physiologic TLESRs.[12]

■ Gastric Distention

Gastric distention (with concomitant shortening of LES length) in patients with GERD may be the result of slow gastric emptying or of aerophagia,[6] an increase in pharyngeal swallowing in an unconscious effort to improve esophageal clearance.

■ Gastroduodenal Reflux

Gastroduodenal reflux, caused perhaps by an incompetent pyloric sphincter, may allow excess amounts of proteolytic enzymes and bile acids into the stomach and eventually into the esophagus.[5] Several investigators have examined the role of refluxed duodenal contents in esophageal injury.

In addition to confirming the well known contribution of acid to esophagitis, Fiorucci and colleagues also demonstrated that mixed acid/alkaline reflux occurred commonly in severe disease.[19] Stein and associates found the complications of GERD to be particularly frequent and severe in patients with both a defective sphincter and increased acid/alkaline exposure (Figure 2.4).[20] Lin and associates have shown that the presence and severity of reflux complications are related to both a mechanically defective sphincter and increased esophageal exposure to excessive reflux of duodenal and gastric juice.[21]

FIGURE 2.4 — THE SEVERITY OF COMPLICATIONS IN PATIENTS WITH GERD AND ACID REFLUX OR ACID/ALKALINE REFLUX WITH AND WITHOUT A MECHANICALLY DEFECTIVE LES

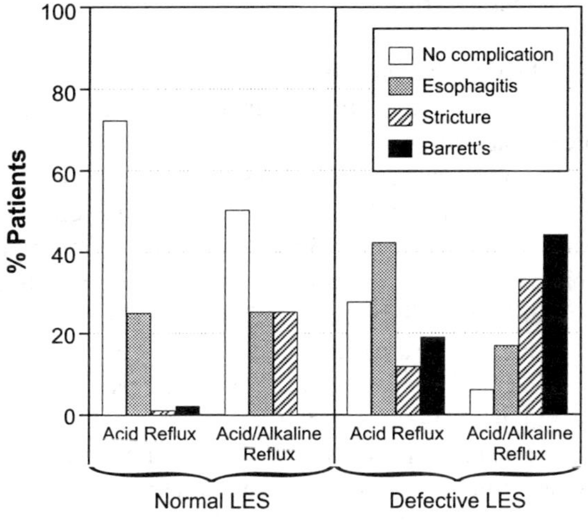

Stein HJ, Barlow AP, DeMeester TR, Hinder RA. Complications of gastroesophageal reflux disease: role of the lower esophageal sphincter, esophageal acid and acid/alkaline exposure, and duodenogastric reflux. *Ann Surg*. 1992;216:41. Reprinted with permission.

However, Gotley and associates[22] found no relationship between severity of esophagitis and the concentration of bile acids in aspirated refluxate and concluded that bile acids (and trypsin) are probably unimportant compared to acid and pepsin. The issue remains unresolved.

■ Gastric Hypersecretion

Gastric hypersecretion can increase esophageal exposure to gastric juice by the physiologic reflux of concentrated acid. In one study of patients with increased esophageal exposure to gastric juice, as measured by 24-hour pH monitoring, 28% were found to secrete excessive amounts of gastric acid.[23] However, a mechanically defective sphincter was more important than gastric hypersecretion in the development of complications of GERD.

■ The Esophageal Tissue Barrier

The esophageal tissue barrier, an integrated complex of anatomic and physiologic components, acts to maintain the integrity of the esophageal mucosa (Figure 2.5).[24] Minor damage to the squamous epithelial cell surface wrought by brief exposure to even highly concentrated gastric acid is rapidly repaired (< 1 hour) by viable epithelial cells, which migrate in amoeba-like fashion over the areas of bared basement membranes.[24]

In GERD, however, the barrier is breached by repeated, prolonged exposure to gastric acid and pepsin and perhaps by refluxed bile salts, and pancreatic enzymes. Surface cells are sloughed and new epithelial cells are produced in the regenerative (basal) zone. With continued exposure to unmodified acid, the surface layer thins and the basal zone widens, with extension of the papillae to the cell surface (Figure 2.6).[1]

Hiatal Hernia

The pathogenic relationship between a hiatal hernia and GERD is somewhat confusing. According to one study, although most patients with moderate to severe esophagitis do have hiatal hernias, the converse is not true: the majority of patients with sliding hiatal hernias do *not* have esophagitis.[2] A later trial, which correlated hiatal hernia and symptomatic esophagitis, found the deciding factor to be the LES pressure.[25] Patients with pressures greater than 12 mm Hg were asymptomatic regardless of whether they had hiatal

FIGURE 2.5 — ESOPHAGEAL DEFENSES: TISSUE RESISTANCE

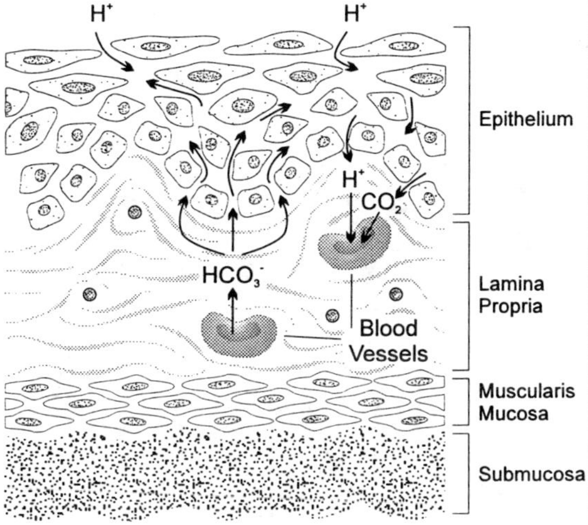

The major postepithelial defense against acid injury is an adequate blood supply. In addition to providing essential nutrients and oxygen for cell metabolism, the blood supply maintains tissue acid-base balance through the delivery of HCO_3^- and removal of H^+ and CO_2. The HCO_3^- contained in the interstitial fluid is important for neutralization of H^+ diffusing through the intercellular space.

hernias. Those with lower LES pressures, with or without hernias, had symptoms.

However, according to a study by Sloan and associates, in the presence of low LES pressure, hiatal hernia does contribute to reflux.[18] The study was designed to examine the recently generated "two sphincter hypothesis" of GEJ incompetence, that is, both the smooth muscle LES and the right diaphragmatic crus encircling the LES serve sphincteric functions. In particular, the

FIGURE 2.6—EFFECTS OF REFLUX ON NORMAL SQUAMOUS MUCOSA

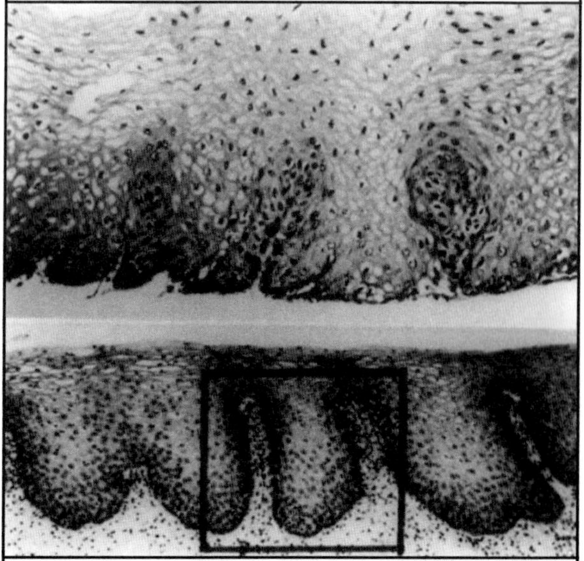

Normal squamous mucosa is shown at the top and the effects of reflux at the bottom. The major changes are (1) thinning of the squamous cell zone, (2) extension of the papillae to the epithelial cell surface (see box), and (3) hypertrophy of the basal cell zone.

Ippoliti A. Inflammatory and infectious esophageal disorders. In: Gitnick G, ed. *Principles and Practice of Gastroenterology and Hepatology*, 2nd ed. Norwalk, Conn: Appleton & Lange; 1994:39. Reprinted with permission.

diaphragm augments the LES during inspiration, coughing or a Mueller maneuver (inspiration against a closed glottis).

What then, asked the investigators, would be the effect of a hiatal hernia on GEJ competence in patients challenged by abrupt increases in intra-abdominal pressure, specifically Valsalva and Mueller maneuvers, leg lifts, and gradual inflation of an abdominal cuff placed below the ribs?[18] The major finding was that susceptibility to gastroesophageal reflux induced by abrupt increases in intra-abdominal pressure was strongly related to both the size of the hiatal hernia and LES pressure (Figure 2.7). In other words, hiatal hernia increases the vulnerability to reflux during periods of concomitant low LES pressure. Therefore, medicines, foods, and habits that reduce LES pressure are more likely to result in reflux in patients with hernias than in those without.

REFERENCES

1. Ippoliti A.Inflammatory and infectious esophageal disorders. In: Gitnick G, ed. *Principles and Practice of Gastroenterology and Hepatology*, 2nd ed. Norwalk, Conn: Appleton & Lange; 1994:37-49.

2. Johnson DA. Medical therapy for gastroesophageal reflux disease. *Am J Med.* 1992;92:88S-97S.

3. Dent J, Holloway RH, Toouli J, Dodds WJ. Mechanisms of lower oesophageal sphincter incompetence in patients with symptomatic gastrooesophageal reflux. *Gut.* 1988; 29:1020-1028.

4. Mittal RK. The sphincter mechanism at the lower end of the esophagus: an overview. *Dysphagia.* 1993;8:347-350.

5. Bozymski EM. Pathophysiology and diagnosis of gastroesophageal reflux disease. *Am J Hosp Pharm.* 1993;50 (suppl 1):S4-S6.

6. Peters JH, DeMeester TR. Gastroesophageal reflux. *Surg Clin North Am.* 1993;73:1119-1144.

7. Dodds WJ, Dent J, Hogan WJ, et al. Mechanisms of gastroesophageal reflux in patients with reflux esophagitis. *N Engl J Med.* 1982;307:1547-1552.

FIGURE 2.7—THE HIATAL HERNIA FACTOR

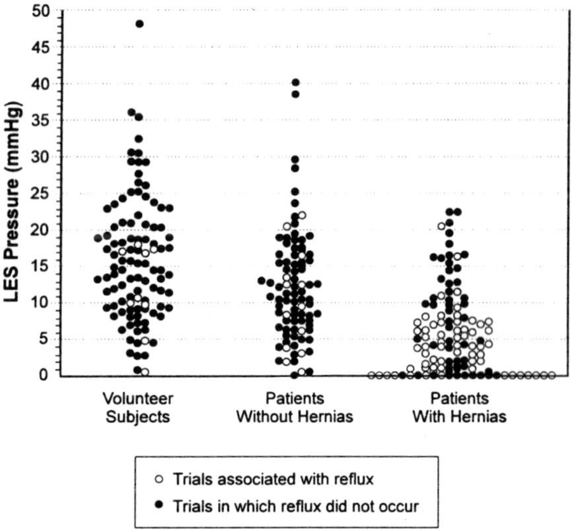

Both LES pressure and hiatal hernia are determinants of susceptibility to reflux reduced by provocative maneuvers. On the one hand, reflux was more likely to occur at a given LES pressure in patients with hernias. On the other hand, reflux was unlikely in the presence of higher LES pressures regardless of hernia status.

Sloan S, Rademaker AW, Kahrilas PJ. Determinants of gastroesophageal junction incompetence: hiatal hernia, lower esophageal sphincter, or both? *Ann Intern Med.* 1992; 117:977-982. Reprinted with permission.

8. Holloway RH, Dent J. Pathophysiology of gastroesophageal reflux. Lower esophageal sphincter dysfunction in gastroesophageal reflux disease. *Gastroenterol Clin Am*. 1990;19:517-535.

9. Bell NJ, Burget D, Howden CW, Wilkinson J, Hunt RH. Appropriate acid suppression for the management of gastro-oesophageal reflux disease. *Digestion*. 1992; 51(suppl 1):59-67.

10. Robertson D, Aldersley M, Shepherd H, Smith CL. Patterns of acid reflux in complicated oesophagitis. *Gut*. 1987;28:1484-1488.

11. Robinson M. Gastroesophageal reflux disease: selecting optimal therapy. *Postgrad Med*. 1994;95:88-102.

12. Morton LS, Fromkes JJ. Gastroesophageal reflux disease: diagnosis and medical therapy. *Geriatrics*. 1993;48:60-66.

13. Kahrilas PJ, Dodds WJ, Hogan WJ. Effect of peristaltic dysfunction on esophageal volume clearance. *Gastroenterology*. 1988;94:73-80.

14. Katz PO, Knuff TE, Benjamin SB, Castell DO. Abnormal esophageal pressures in reflux esophagitis: cause or effect? *Am J Gastroenterol*. 1986;81:744-746.

15. Triadafilopoulos G, Castillo T. Nonpropulsive esophageal contractions and gastroesophageal reflux. *Am J Gastroenterol*. 1991;86:153-159.

16. Crozier RE, Glick ME, Gibb SP, Ellis FH Jr, Veerman JM. Acid-provoked esophageal spasm as a cause of noncardiac chest pain. *Am J Gastroenterol*. 1991;86:1576-1580.

17. Helm JF, Dodds WJ, Hogan WJ. Salivary response to esophageal acid in normal subjects and patients with reflux esophagitis. *Gastroenterology*. 1987;93:1393-1397.

18. Sloan S, Rademaker AW, Kahrilas PJ. Determinants of gastroesophageal junction incompetence: hiatal hernia, lower esophageal sphincter, or both? *Ann Intern Med*. 1992;117:977-982.

19. Fiorucci S, Santucci L, Chiucchiú S, Morelli A. Gastric acidity and gastroesophageal reflux patterns in patients with esophagitis. *Gastroenterology*. 1992;103:855-861.

20. Stein HJ, Barlow AD, DeMeester TR, Hinder RA. Complications of gastroesophageal reflux disease. Role of the lower esophageal sphincter, esophageal acid and acid/alkaline exposure, and duodenogastric reflux. *Ann Surg*. 1992;216:35-43.

21. Lin KM, Ueda RK, Hinder RA, Stein HJ, DeMeester TR. Etiology and importance of alkaline esophageal reflux. *Am J Surg*. 1991;162:553-557.

22. Gotley DC, Morgan AP, Ball D, Owen RW, Cooper MJ. Composition of gastro-oesophageal refluxate. *Gut*. 1991; 32:1093-1099.

23. Barlow AP, DeMeester TR, Ball CS, Eypasch EP. The significance of the gastric secretory state in gastroesophageal reflux disease. *Arch Surg*. 1989;124:937-940.

24. Orlando RC. Reflux esophagitis. In: Yamada T, Alpers DH, Owyang C, Powell DW, Silverstein FE, eds. *Textbook of Gastroenterology*.Philadelphia, Pa: Lippincott; 1991:1123.

25. Cohen S, Harris LD. Does hiatus hernia affect competence of the gastroesophageal sphincter? *N Engl J Med*. 1971;284:1053-1056.

PART 2

DIAGNOSIS OF GASTROESOPHAGEAL REFLUX DISEASE

3 Symptoms

The symptoms of gastroesophageal reflux disease (GERD) are diverse and often suggestive of a number of other, sometimes more serious, diseases (Table 3.1). The typical manifestations are:

- Heartburn
- Acid regurgitation
- Hypersalivation
- Nonobstructive dysphagia.

3

Heartburn

Heartburn, a burning, substernal pain traveling up the esophagus toward the pharynx,[1] is the most common symptom of GERD.[2] It most often occurs:

- 30 to 60 minutes after meals[3]
- On reclining after food intake
- With certain body positions.[4]

Approximately one-tenth of the U.S. population experiences heartburn daily; a third, once a month; and a quarter of women have it throughout pregnancy.[5]

Acid Regurgitation

Regurgitation of digestive juice to the throat often accompanies heartburn. An occasional patient may refer to regurgitation as vomiting; a differential clue is that it occurs without effort and is often precipitated by a postural change.[6]

TABLE 3.1 — SYMPTOMS OF GERD
Typical • Heartburn • Acid regurgitation • Hypersalivation • Odynophagia • Unobstructive dysphagia **Atypical** • Angina-like chest pain • Cough • Nonallergic asthma • Chronic bronchitis (?) • Hoarseness • Globus • Pneumonia (aspiration)
Modified from: Anggiansah A, Owen WA, Owen WJ. The investigation and management of gastro-oesophageal reflux disease. *BJCP.* 1993; 47:256-261; and, Ippoliti A. Inflammatory and infectious esophageal disorders. In: Gitnick G, ed. *Principles and Practice of Gastroenterology and Hepatology*, 2nd ed. Norwalk, Conn: Appleton & Lange; 1994: 40-41. Reprinted with permission.

Hypersalivation

Hypersalivation, or water brash, another common symptom, may be a protective response to refluxed acid.[7] Odynophagia and esophageal sensitivity to hot liquids or alcohol, also suggest GERD.[6]

Nonobstructive Dysphagia

Nonobstructive dysphagia is reported in up to 45% of reflux patients.[8] Ambulatory manometric studies of 27 GERD patients revealed more meal-related swallows followed by inadequate peristaltic waves in the 16 patients (59%) with dysphagia.[8] Thus a peristaltic abnormality may be responsible for this relatively common symptom in patients with reflux. However, dysphagia warrants careful diagnosis since it often indicates esophageal stricture or Barrett's esophagus (Figure 3.1).

Atypical Symptoms

The major atypical symptoms of GERD are:

- Chest pain
- Respiratory symptoms
- Hoarseness.

■ Chest Pain

3

According to an early study by Bennett and Atkinson, 23% of patients admitted as emergencies with clinically suspected myocardial infarction were eventually found to have alimentary tract disease, mostly esophagitis.[9] More recently, Anggiansah and colleagues found GERD to be associated with noncardiac chest pain in 38% of patients referred from the department of cardiology in one hospital and originally thought to have angina.[10]

■ Respiratory Symptoms

Respiratory symptoms are increasingly seen in reflux disease.[11] Microaspiration of refluxate that reaches the hypopharynx appears to be the principal mechanism.[12] The resulting symptoms of cough, choking, and even recurrent pneumonia often evade initial association with GERD. Repair of respiratory epithelium lost secondary to aspiration can take as long as seven days, during which the acid-induced irritation gives rise to a chronic cough.[13] Thus studies during that period of repair may find no relationship between the cough and reflux episodes.[13] The cause of aspiration seems to lie primarily in abnormal lower esophageal

FIGURE 3.1—DIFFERENTIAL DIAGNOSIS OF DYSPHAGIA

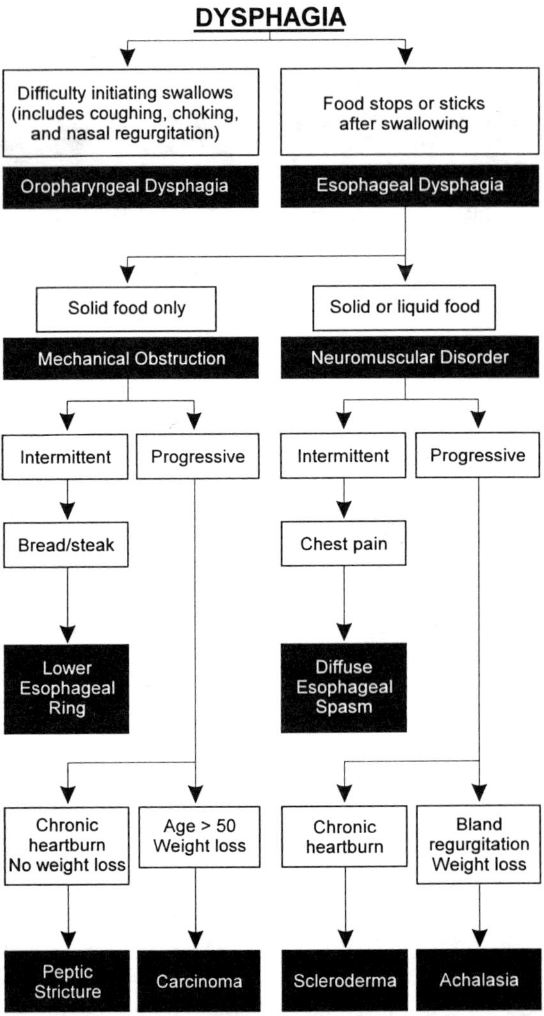

Modified from: *Cecil Essentials of Medicine*, 3rd ed. Andreoli TE, Bennett JC, Carpenter CCJ, Plum F, Smith LH Jr, eds. Philadelphia, Pa: WB Saunders Company; 1993:284. Reprinted with permission.

sphincter (LES) function and esophageal clearance, which are more common in GERD patients who have pulmonary complications.[14]

Pulmonary symptoms are particularly common in older patients, in whom radiographic changes on chest x-rays (parenchymal scarring and pleural thickening) may be the only indicators of GERD.[15]

Whether chronic bronchitis can be a consequence of GERD is unclear.[2] It has been suggested that reflux can induce bronchial constriction either by aspiration or by stimulation of vagal efferent fibers to the lung. In patients with adult-onset nonallergic asthma, particularly those with nocturnal wheezing, reflux should be considered.

■ Hoarseness

Occasionally, hoarseness may be a major manifestation.[16] How the physiologic factors in GERD contribute to this laryngeal manifestation is unknown. Prolonged pH monitoring in patients with hoarseness or laryngeal cancer has demonstrated abnormal acid refluxate in the distal esophagus, but not consistently in the pharyngeal region (Figure 3.2).[16-18] Associated complaints include:

- Sore throat
- Bad breath
- A full sensation in the neck (globus).[6]

FIGURE 3.2—PHARYNGOESOPHAGEAL pH MONITORING

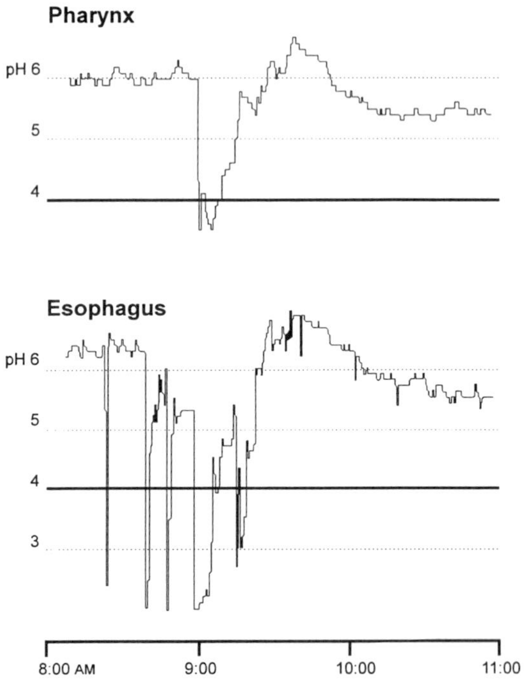

Among 15 patients with chronic hoarseness and laryngeal lesions suggestive of acid irritation who underwent dual-pharyngoesophageal pH monitoring, 12 had abnormal esophageal pH studies. Three of the 12 also showed definite pharyngeal reflux seen here beginning at 9 AM with its concomitant drop in esophageal pH to below 4.0.

Wiener GJ, Koufman JA, Wu WC, et al. Chronic hoarseness secondary to gastroesophageal reflux disease: documentation with 24-h ambulatory pH monitoring. *Am J Gastroenterol*. 1989;84:1506. Reprinted with permission.

REFERENCES

1. Bozymski EM. Pathophysiology and diagnosis of gastroesophageal reflux disease. *Am J Hosp Pharm*. 1993;50 (suppl 1):S4-S6.

2. Ippoliti A. Inflammatory and infectious esophageal disorders. In: Gitnick G, ed. *Principles and Practice of Gastroenterology and Hepatology*, 2nd ed. Norwalk, Conn: Appleton & Lange; 1994:37-49.

3. Tierney LM, McPhee SJ, Papadakis MA. *Current Medical Diagnosis and Treatment*. Norwalk, Conn: Appleton & Lange; 1994:479-482.

4. Johnson DA. Medical therapy for gastroesophageal reflux disease. *Am J Med*. 1992;92(suppl 5A):88S-97S.

5. Richter JE. A critical review of current medical therapy for gastroesophageal reflux disease. *J Clin Gastroenterol*. 1986;8 (suppl 1):72-80.

6. Anggiansah A, Owen WA, Owen WJ. The investigation and management of gastro-oesophageal reflux disease. *Br J Clin Pract*. 1993;47:256-261.

7. Helm JF, Dodds WJ, Homan WJ. Salivary response to esophageal acid in normal subjects and patients with reflux esophagitis. *Gastroenterology*. 1987;93:1393-1397.

8. Singh S, Stein HJ, DeMeester TR, Hinder RA. Nonobstructive dysphagia in gastroesophageal reflux disease: a study with combined ambulatory pH and motility monitoring. *Am J Gastroenterol*. 1992;87:562-567.

9. Bennett JR, Atkinson M. The differentiation between oesophageal and cardiac pain. *Lancet*. 1966;2:1123-1127.

10. Anggiansah A, Chambers J, Cooke R, Bright NF, Sumboonnanonda K, Owen WJ. Non-cardiac chest pain (NCCP)—is it gastro-oesophageal reflux? *Gut*. 1991;32:A1212-A1213. Abstract.

11. Clouse RE, Chokshi HR. The esophagus. In: Gitnick G, ed. *Current Gastroenterology*, vol. 14. St. Louis, Mo: Mosby–Year Book, Inc; 1994:1-28.

12. Pellegrini CA, DeMeester TR, Johnson LF, Skinner DB. Gastroesophageal reflux and pulmonary aspiration: incidence, functional abnormality, and results of surgical therapy. *Surgery*. 1979;86:110-119.

13. Peters JH, DeMeester TR. Gastroesophageal reflux. *Surg Clin North Am*. 1993;73:1119-1144.

14. Patti MG, Debas HT, Pellegrini CA. Esophageal manometry and 24-hour pH monitoring in the diagnosis of pulmonary aspiration secondary to gastroesophageal reflux. *Am J Surg*. 1992;163:401-406.

15. Räihä I, Manner R, Hietanen E, Hartiala J, Sourander L. Radiographic pulmonary changes of gastro-oesophageal reflux disease in elderly patients. *Age Ageing*. 1992;21:250-255.

16. Robinson M. Gastroesophageal reflux disease. Selecting optimal therapy. *Postgrad Med*. 1994;95:88-102.

17. Katz PO, Bishop SG, Lumpkin SMM. Chronic dysphonia secondary to gastroesophageal reflux (GER): diagnosis with continuous dual-ambulatory pH monitoring (CDA pHM). *Gastroenterology*. 1988;94:A219. Abstract.

18. Wiener GJ, Koufman JA, Wu WC, Cooper JB, Richter JE, Castell DO. Chronic hoarseness secondary to gastroesophageal reflux disease: documentation with 24-h ambulatory pH monitoring. *Am J Gastroenterol*. 1989;84:1503-1508.

4 Diagnosis

An extensive diagnostic workup is not indicated in every patient with suspected gastroesophageal reflux disease (GERD), particularly in young persons with classical symptoms of heartburn and regurgitation. If the medical history reveals that symptoms are either postprandial or associated with abrupt or extreme postural changes (such as strenuous exercise), a trial of empiric treatment is appropriate.[1,2]

For a young patient with classical presumptive diagnosis, change of habits related to symptoms, use of antacids (if they have not already been tried), or brief trials of two pharmaceutical agents that act differently to suppress acid secretion are worthwhile: a histamine$_2$-receptor antagonist (H_2-RA) or an acid pump inhibitor (API), also called a proton pump inhibitor (PPI).

In the presence of an atypical or mixed syndrome, further investigation is generally necessary. A diagnosis of GERD does not rule out concomitant respiratory or cardiac disease nor, for that matter, do either of those conditions rule out GERD.

Atypical or refractory symptoms or concomitant weight loss and anemia should always raise the index of suspicion (Figure 3.1).[2,3]

Objective diagnostic procedures are useful to quantify the content and severity of disease and to address three questions:

- Does reflux exist?
- Is acid reflux responsible for the patient's symptoms?
- Has reflux led to esophageal damage?

Currently available diagnostic tests include:

- Prolonged, usually 24-hour, pH monitoring
- Manometry of the lower esophageal sphincter (LES)
- Manometry of the esophageal body
- Endoscopy, with biopsy
- Barium esophagogram
- Prolonged motility monitoring
- Acid perfusion (Bernstein) test
- Radionuclide studies.

Prolonged pH Monitoring

The gold standard for measuring acid exposure, 24-hour pH monitoring, is indicated in the following circumstances:[1,2]

- When patients present with atypical symptoms, such as noncardiac chest pain
- When symptoms do not respond to trials of conventional therapy
- In preparation for antireflux surgery.

Ambulatory monitoring is performed by passing a small microelectrode pH probe transnasally to 5 cm above the upper border of the LES.[4] Data from the probe are collected in a small portable box that the patient wears on a waistband while continuing his or her activities at home and work.[1] Monitoring for a 24-hour period allows measurement of the effect of various physiologic activities on reflux over a complete circadian cycle.[4] Diagnostic parameters include:

- Quantitation of the actual time the esophageal mucosa is exposed to gastric juice
- Measurement of the esophageal ability to clear refluxed acid
- Correlation of reflux episodes with symptoms.[5]

A diary or the event marker on the pH monitor is used to record meal, bed, and getting-up times, as well as the occurrence of symptoms, all of which are important in determining the temporal relationship between symptoms and acid reflux.[1] This relationship is particularly useful for determining whether atypical symptoms, such as chest pain, cough, or wheezing, are secondary to acid reflux.

Computerized analysis of pH monitoring produces reports on six variables in pH status over 24 hours (Table 4.1). False negative pH results may occur as a result of duodenogastric reflux or of gastric hypochlorhydria.[1] In such circumstances, dual-channel pH studies that use gastric and esophageal probes to simultaneously measure will help identify the problem.

TABLE 4.1 — VARIABLES MEASURED DURING ESOPHAGEAL PH MONITORING

- Number of reflux episodes
- Number of reflux episodes lasting more than 5 minutes
- Longest reflux episode
- Percentage time pH less than 4
- Percentage time pH less than 4 in a supine position
- Percentage time pH less than 4 in an upright position

Anggiansah A, Owen WA, Owen WJ. The investigation and management of gastro-oesophageal reflux disease. *BJCP*. 1993;47:256-261. Reprinted with permission.

4

Other causes of increased alkaline exposure (in the pH 7 or 8 range) include:[4]

- Improper calibration of the pH recorder
- The presence of dental infection, which increases salivary pH
- The presence of esophageal obstruction, which results in static pools of saliva with an increase in pH secondary to bacterial overgrowth.

Placement of an additional electrode in the proximal esophagus or pharynx also can be helpful in patients with chronic cough, hoarseness, or symptoms of pulmonary aspiration.[6] If refluxed material is reaching as far as the pharynx and a temporal relationship is indicated between reflux episodes and onset of symptoms, GERD is the most likely cause of the patient's complaints.

Prolonged pH monitoring has a sensitivity of 88% and a specificity of 98% given strict adherence to:

- Directions for probe placement
- Calibration of the pH recorder
- Interpretation of results.[1]

Comparison of 24-hour pH monitoring with other common diagnostic tests is seen in Figure 4.1.

Manometry of the Lower Esophageal Sphincter

The most accurate method for quantitation of the sphincter's resistance to the reflux of gastric juice, LES manometry permits determination of LES pressure and length, both abdominal and overall.

A catheter with four to eight radial side holes is introduced intranasally into the stomach.[7] As the catheter is withdrawn through the gastroesophageal junction, for each level of pullback, radially measured pressures are plotted around an axis, representing gastric baseline pressure (Figure 4.2). The respiratory inversion point (the level at which the positive deflections in the pressure curve caused by inspiration within the abdomen changed to negative within the chest) was used to identify the intra-abdominal portion of the sphincter. Three-dimensional images of the sphincter are created on a computer screen and rotated to allow inspection for asymmetry. The volume circumscribed

FIGURE 4.1—DIAGNOSTIC TESTS FOR GERD

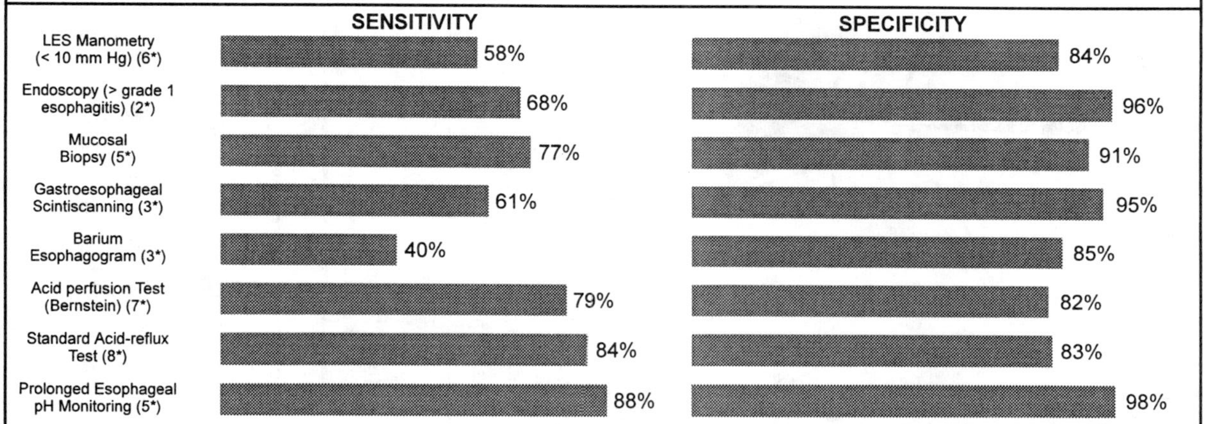

* Number of studies from which sensitivity and specificity were calculated.

DeMeester TR, Stein HJ. Gastroesophageal reflux disease. In: Moody FG, ed. *Surgical Treatment of Digestive Disease*. 2nd ed. Chicago, Ill: Year Book Medical Publishers, Inc; 1986:67. Reprinted with permission.

FIGURE 4.2—COMPUTERIZED 3-DIMENSIONAL IMAGING OF LES

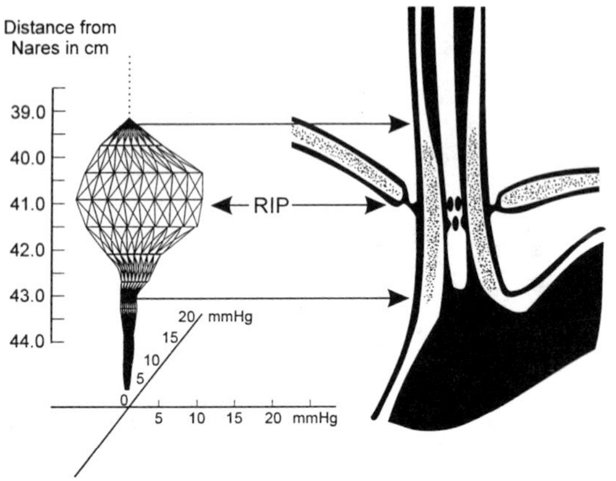

A catheter with four to eight radial side holes is withdrawn through the gastroesophageal junction. For each level of the pullback, the radially measured pressures are plotted around an axis, representing gastric baseline pressure. When a stepwise pullback technique is used, the respiratory inversion point (RIP) can be identified.

Stein HJ, DeMeester TR, Naspetti R, Jamieson J, Perry RE. Three-dimensional imaging of the lower esophageal sphincter in gastroesophageal reflux disease. *Ann Surg*. 1991;214:377. Reprinted with permission.

by that image integrates pressures exerted over the sphincter's length and around its circumference into one number. This number represents sphincter resistance to the reflux of gastric contents.

Manometry of the Esophageal Body

This measurement is essential to assess esophageal propulsive force, which depends on peristaltic contractions.[4] Using simultaneous fluoroscopy and manometry of the esophageal body, Kahrilas and associates found that the peristaltic amplitudes of contraction required for invariable bolus clearance were 16 mm Hg in the proximal esophagus and 30 mm Hg to 40 mm Hg distally.[8]

Ambulatory 24-Hour Esophageal/pH Manometry

The recent advance of ambulatory 24-hour esophageal motility monitoring allows assessment of esophageal body function over an entire circadian cycle under a variety of physiologic conditions.[9] Frequency of ineffective contractions can be quantified based on approximately 1000 contractions monitored while patients are sleeping, awake, or eating.[4]

Simultaneous esophageal/pH monitoring permits assessment of the esophageal body's direct response to a spontaneous reflux episode.[4] Initial results show that acid clearance after a reflux episode depends on the frequency of primary (pharyngeally-induced) effective contractions. This response appears to be compromised in patients with severe esophagitis or Barrett's esophagus, because of the loss of muscular contraction amplitude in the esophageal body, caused by the inflammatory process.

Endoscopy With Biopsy

Endoscopy is the most useful of the available tests for assessing esophagitis, as well as complications such as esophageal stricture and Barrett's esophagus. Indications for endoscopy are:

- A brief history of symptoms in older patients (> 50 years)
- Associated weight loss

- Dysphagia or bleeding
- Failure to respond to an H_2-RA.[1]

Direct visualization of the esophagus may also be helpful to allay a patient's concern, and sometimes a clinician's anxiety, about possible malignancy.[1] Biopsy is generally called for in any but an endoscopically normal esophagus.

Barium Esophagoscopy

The radiographic demonstration of gastroesophageal reflux depends on the fluoroscopic observation of barium entering the esophagus from the stomach (Figure 4.3).[10] The magnitude of reflux is determined by noting whether the retrograde flow of barium extends into the lower, middle, or upper esophagus.

In adults with symptomatic GERD, radiographic reflux of barium is observed with variable success in 10% to 15% of patients. Conversely, few asymptomatic patients will demonstrate spontaneous reflux radiographically. Although stress maneuvers may further enhance the demonstration of reflux, they also reduce its specificity.

Furthermore, the water siphon test (positive when barium refluxes into the esophagus while the patient swallows water) is of questionable value for accurately separating patients with GERD from healthy subjects.

In short, in half or more of symptomatic patients, spontaneous gastrointestinal reflux of barium is not observed.

Barium studies are more useful for evaluating motor function, diagnosing hiatal hernia and esophageal diverticulae, and detecting complications of GERD, such as esophageal strictures and ulceration (Figure 4.4).[10]

FIGURE 4.3—BARIUM X-RAY SHOWING REFLUX IN PATIENT WITH SCLERODERMA

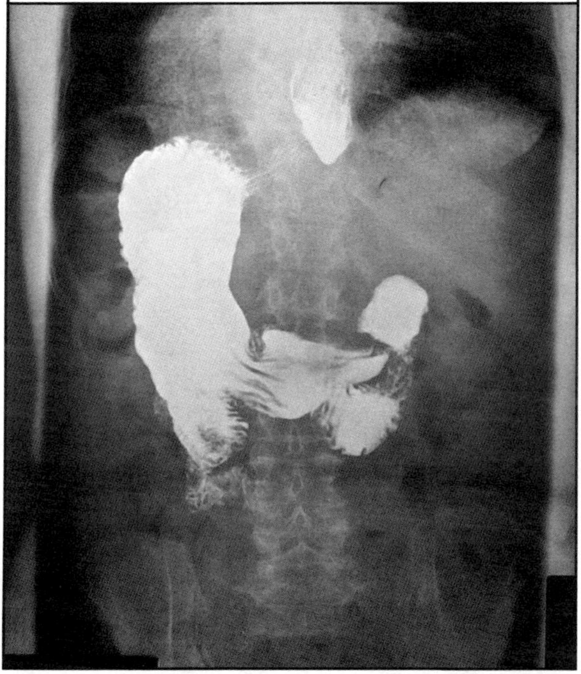

4

Acid Perfusion (Bernstein) Test

The acid perfusion test is used to determine whether a patient's atypical symptoms are acid-induced. The tip of a nasogastric tube is positioned 35 cm from the nares and the esophagus is perfused with saline at a rate of 120 drops/min for 15 minutes, followed by 0.1 N HCl (at the same rate) for 30 minutes.[11] If symptoms occur during acid perfusion, the saline regimen is repeated. Reproduction of the patient's symptoms with acid and relief with saline represents a positive result.

FIGURE 4.4—BARIUM SWALLOW OF PATIENT WITH ESOPHAGEAL STRICTURE

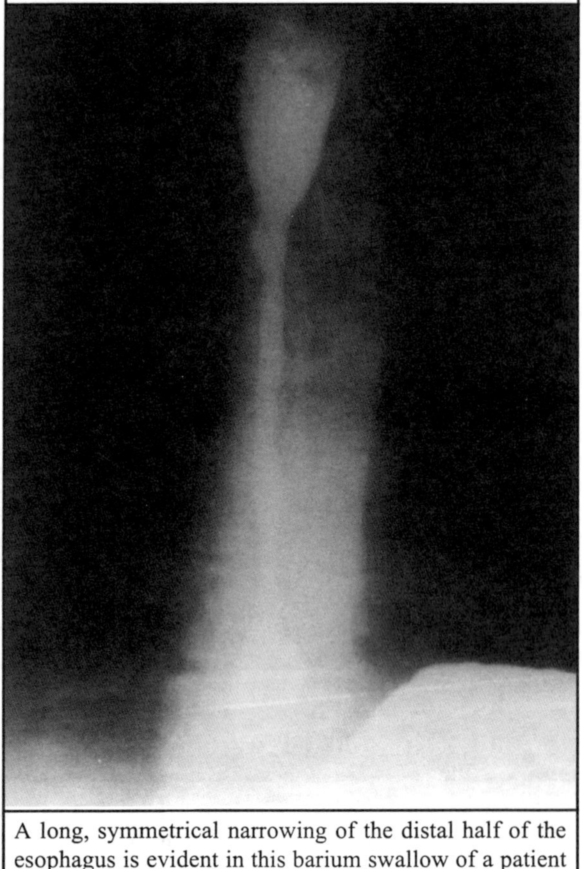

A long, symmetrical narrowing of the distal half of the esophagus is evident in this barium swallow of a patient with esophageal stricture.

Ippoliti A. Inflammatory and infectious esophageal disorders. In:Gitnick G, ed. *Principles and Practice of Gastroenterology and Hepatology*, 2nd ed. Norwalk, Conn: Appleton & Lange; 1994:41. Reprinted with permission.

The test is positive in the majority of patients with typical symptoms of reflux (80% to 90%). Unfortunately, however, 10% to 15% of healthy, asymptomatic controls also test positive. Moreover, some patients with atypical symptoms have equivocal responses regardless of other evidence of acid-induced disease.

The Bernstein test should be used with caution in patients with known coronary disease since it can increase cardiac work and induce angina symptoms.[12]

Radionuclide Studies

Dynamic radionuclide imaging with agents such as technetium Tc 99m sulfur colloid potentially offers a convenient, noninvasive technique for detecting GERD.[13] In a study involving 15 patients with the severest forms of GERD, however, Jenkins and associates found that although reflux is accurately detected by scintigraphy, the intermittent occurrence of reflux episodes limits the test's sensitivity.[13] They conclude that this technique may be more applicable to infants and children in whom more invasive tests are difficult to perform and poorly tolerated.

4

REFERENCES

1. Anggiansah A, Owen WA, Owen WJ. The investigation and management of gastro-oesophageal reflux disease. *Br J Clin Prac*. 1993;47:256-261.

2. Morton LS, Fromkes JJ. Gastroesophageal reflux disease: diagnosis and medical therapy. *Geriatrics*. 1993;48:60-66.

3. Bozymski EM. Pathophysiology and diagnosis of gastroesophageal reflux disease. *Am J Hosp Pharm*. 1993;50 (suppl 1):S4-S6.

4. Peters JH, DeMeester TR. Gastroesophageal reflux. *Surg Clin North Am*. 1993;73:1119-1143.

5. DeMeester TR, Wang CI, Wernly JA, et al. Technique, indications and clinical use of 24-hour esophageal pH monitoring. *J Thorac Cardiovasc Surg*. 1980;79:656-670.

6. Jacob P, Kahrilas PJ, Herzon G. Proximal esophageal pH-metry in patients with "reflux laryngitis." *Gastroenterology*. 1991;100:305-310.

7. Stein HJ, DeMeester TR, Naspetti R, Jamieson J, Perry RE. Three-dimensional imaging of the lower esophageal sphincter in gastroesophageal reflux disease. *Ann Surg*. 1991;214:374-384.

8. Kahrilas PJ, Dodds WJ, Hogan WJ. Effect of peristaltic dysfunction on esophageal volume clearance. *Gastroenterology*. 1988;94:73-80.

9. Stein HJ, DeMeester TR, Singh S. Circadian esophageal motor function in patients with unobstructive dysphagia and normal esophageal acid exposure. *Gastroenterology*. 1991;100:A168. Abstract.

10. Ott DJ, Dodds WJ, Wu WC, Gelfand DW, Hogan WJ, Stewart ET. Current status of radiology in evaluating gastroesophageal reflux disease. *J Clin Gastroenterol*. 1982; 4:365-375.

11. Ippoliti A. Inflammatory and infectious esophageal disorders. In: Gitnick G, ed. *Principles and Practice of Gastroenterology and Hepatology*, 2nd ed. Norwalk, Conn: Appleton & Lange; 1994:19.

12. Mellow MH, Simpson AG, Watt L, Schoolmeester L, Haye OL. Esophageal acid perfusion in coronary artery disease. Induction of myocardial ischemia. *Gastroenterology*. 1983;85:306-312.

13. Jenkins AF, Cowan RJ, Richter JE. Gastroesophageal scintigraphy: is it a sensitive screening test for gastroesophageal reflux disease? *J Clin Gastroenterol*. 1985;7:127-131.

5 Complications

The major complications of gastroesophageal reflux disease (GERD) are erosive/ulcerative esophagitis, esophageal stricture, and Barrett's esophagus, all of which result from the damage inflicted by gastric juice on the esophageal mucosa and changes caused by subsequent repair and fibrosis.[1]

Esophagitis

For the purposes of this book, esophagitis is graded from 1 to 4 on endoscopy (Figure 5.1)[1]; other classifications exist:

- *Grade 1*—Esophageal redness without erosions. The sensitivity of endoscopic detection varies with the observer; biopsy evidence of mucosal infiltration with polymorphonuclear cells, lymphocytes, eosinophils, and balloon cells[2] is confirmatory
- *Grade 2*—Linear erosions paved with granulation tissue that bleeds easily when touched
- *Grade 3*—Erosions coalesce, leaving islands of epithelium, the so-called "cobblestone" esophagus
- *Grade 4*—The presence of a stricture, which can be assessed by the ease, or difficulty, in passing a 36-Fr endoscope; deep ulcer.

Bleeding may be a complication of erosive esophagitis.[3] (Anemia may be a sign of chronic blood loss.)

FIGURE 5.1—ENDOSCOPIC SERIES OF ESOPHAGITIS GRADES

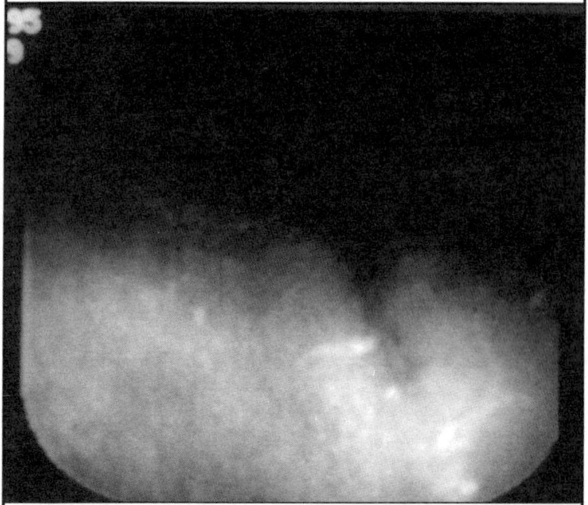

Grade 2 esophagitis, mid-esophagus

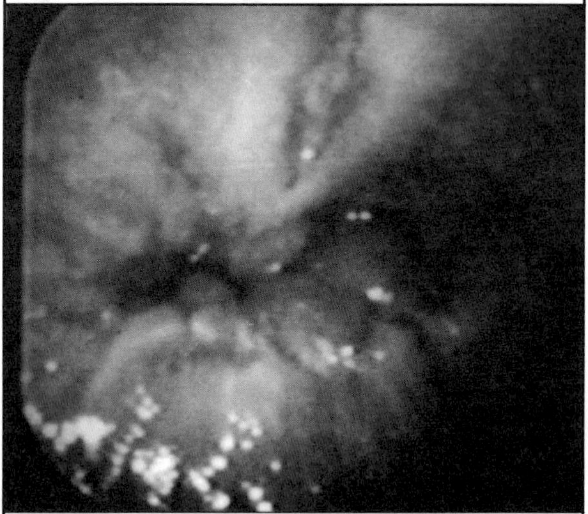

Grade 2 esophagitis, LES region

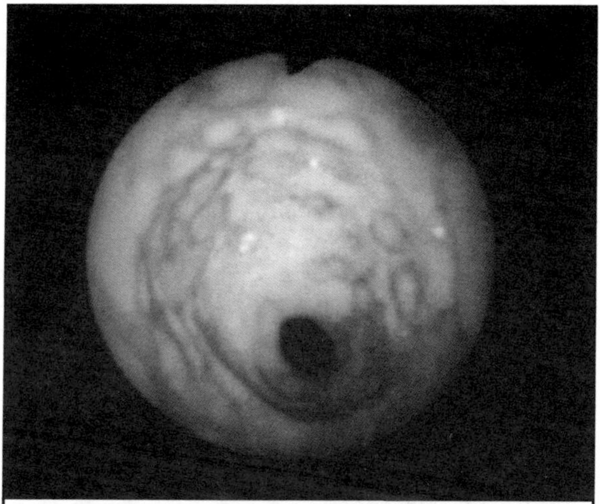

Grade 3 esophagitis

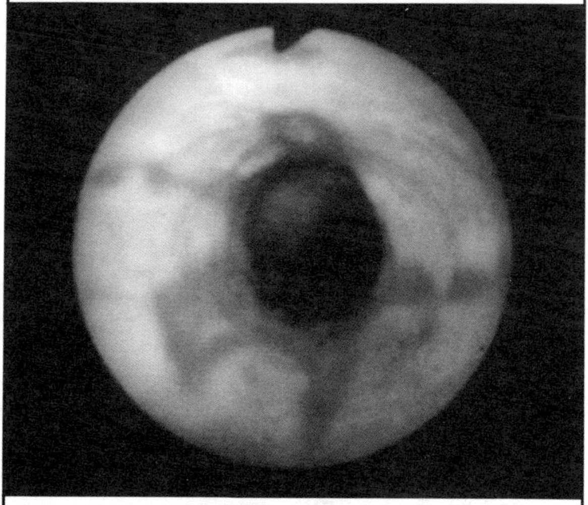

Grade 4 esophagitis

Endoscopic pictures from the esophagus; series showing esophagitis grades 2 through 4.

Photographs courtesy of Wilfred M. Weinstein, MD.

5

Esophageal Strictures

Strictures associated with severe erosive esophagitis develop from submucosal, and eventually intramural, fibrosis. They begin in the gastroesophageal junction (GEJ) and extend proximally for variable distances.[4] The average lesion is 1 cm to 2 cm long[3] and may be as narrow as 2 mm to 3 mm.[5] An estimated 10% of patients treated for GERD have peptic stricture, yet 25% of patients with stricture report no previous symptoms of GERD.[6] Presenting complaints of stricture include:

- Dysphagia
- Odynophagia
- Food impaction.[3]

Most GERD-induced strictures are actually complications of Barrett's esophagus, however. Fibrotic strictures should not be ascribed to reflux esophagitis without hard evidence of prolonged repetitive exposure to gastric juice. In patients with normal acid exposure, stricture may be secondary to a drug-induced chemical injury, the result of a capsule or tablet lodged in the distal esophagus (Figure 5.2, Table 5.1).[7]

Barrett's Esophagus

A recent population-based study revealed an autopsy-estimated prevalence of Barrett's esophagus of 376 per 100,000, a greater than 16-fold increase from that of the 22.6 per 100,000 clinically diagnosed cases.[8]

Patients with GERD are considered to have a greater incidence of Barrett's esophagus compared to others undergoing endoscopy.[9]

Difficulty in visualizing the squamocolumnar junction at its normal location and the presence of a redder, more luxuriant mucosa than normally seen in the lower

FIGURE 5.2 — SCHEMATIC OF DRUG-INDUCED ESOPHAGEAL STRICTURE

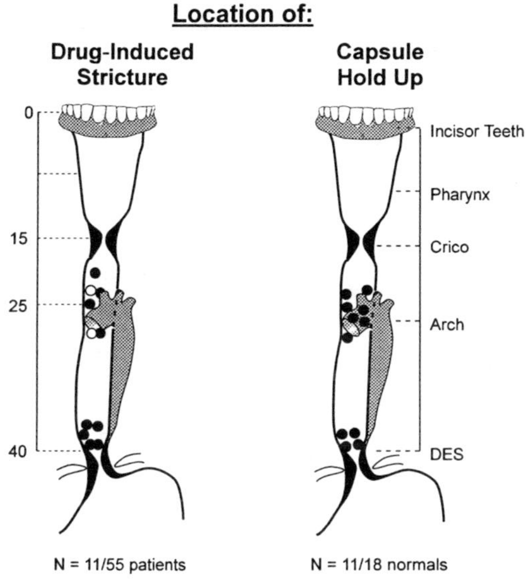

Schematic drawing of the esophagus showing that the site of capsule lodgment in 11 volunteers after a 15-mL water chaser was similar to the location of drug-induced stricture in 11 patients.

Modified from: Bonavina L, DeMeester TR, McChesney L, Schwizer W, Albertucci M, Bailey RT. Drug-induced esophageal strictures. *Ann Surg*. 1987;206:180. Reprinted with permission.

esophagus should arouse suspicion of Barrett's esophagus (Figure 5.3 and 5.4).[1]

In the majority of studies, Barrett's esophagus is defined as specialized columnar epithelium (SCE) 3 cm above the GEJ.[9] To determine the prevalence of shorter-segment changes, Zeroogian and associates obtained

TABLE 5.1—CAUSE AND TREATMENT OF DRUG-INDUCED ESOPHAGEAL STRICTURES

Patient	Medication	Period of Exposure	Therapy	Result
1	Potassium chloride	3 mos	Dilatation with progressive difficulty, resection and colon interposition	Good (8 yrs)
2	Potassium chloride	2 wks	Dilatation (N = 45)	Good (3 yrs)
3	Doxycycline hyclate	1 yr	Dilatation (N = 1)	Good (10 mos)
4	Acetylsalicylic acid	1 wk	Dilatation (N = 1)	Good (20 mos)
5	Tetracycline hydrochloride	6 mos	Dilatation (N = 4)	Good (2 yrs)
6	Potassium chloride	1 yr	Unable to dilate, colon bypass	Good (6 yrs)
7	Ascorbic acid	2 mos	Perforation during dilatation, resection and colon interposition	Good (18 mos)

8	Phenytoin sodium	6 yrs	Dilatation with progressive difficulty, sleeve resection	Induced gastroesophageal reflux (5 yrs)
9	Doxycycline hyclate	1 yr	Dilatation with progressive difficulty, excision fibrous ring and esophageal myotomy, colon bypass	Good (2 yrs)
10	Acetylsalicylic acid	1 wk	Dilatation (N = 1)	Good (9 mos)
11	Quinidine	4 mos	Dilatation (N = 1)	Good (3 mos)

Bonavina L, DeMeester TR, McChesney L, et al. Drug-induced esophageal strictures. *Ann Surg*. 1987;206:176. Reprinted with permission.

5

FIGURE 5.3—ENDOSCOPIC VIEW OF SUSPECTED BARRETT'S ESOPHAGUS

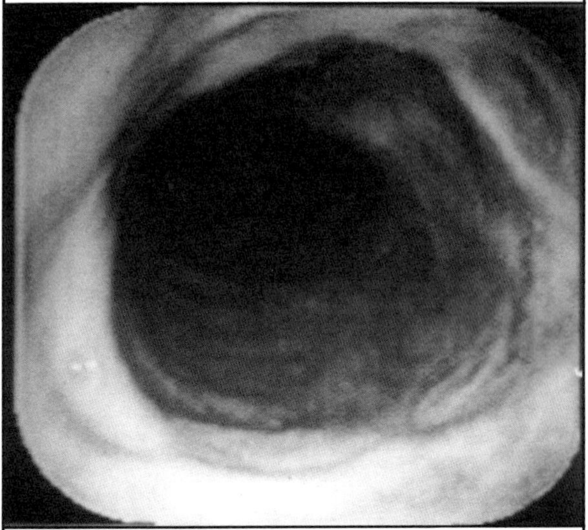

Gastrointestinal Pathology and Its Clinical Implications. Lewin KJ, Riddell RH, Weinstein WM, eds. New York/Tokyo: Igaku Shoin Publishers; 1992. Reprinted with permission.

biopsy specimens from consenting patients undergoing endoscopy at one hospital.[10]

Among 90 patients not known to have Barrett's, the investigators found SCE lining greater than 2 cm of the distal esophagus in only two (2.2%), whereas 18 patients (20%) had similar changes less than or equal to 2 cm above the junction (short-segment Barrett's).[10]

Furthermore, 7 of the 18 patients had no endoscopic signs nor any symptomatic evidence of esophagitis; and four of the seven had no histologic evidence of esophageal inflammation.

Strictures that complicate Barrett's esophagus develop at the site of maximal injury, the interface be-

FIGURE 5.4—HISTOLOGIC SECTION OF BARRETT'S ESOPHAGUS

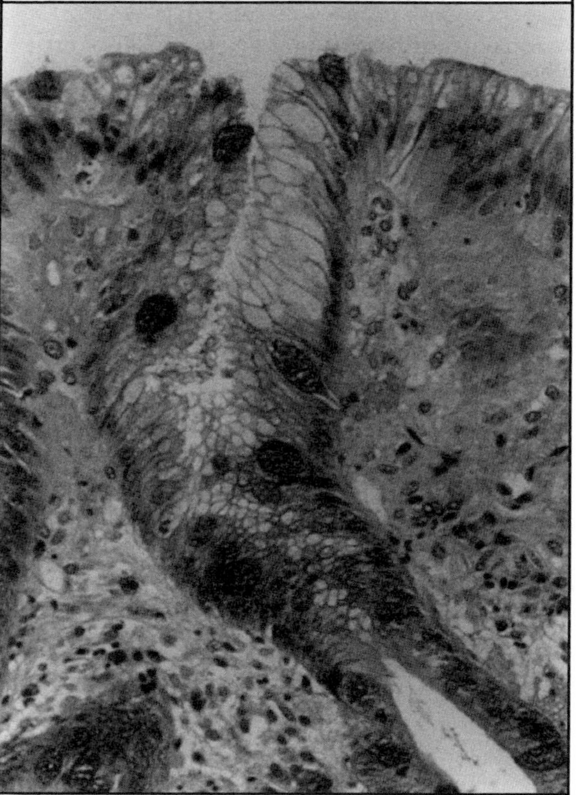

Gastrointestinal Pathology and Its Clinical Implications. Lewin KJ, Riddell RH, Weinstein WM, eds. New York/Tokyo: Igaku Shoin Publishers; 1992. Reprinted with permission.

tween the columnar and squamous epithelium.[1] As the columnar epithelium advances into the area of esophagitis, refluxate may spill over to the proximal mucosa, and the stricture moves progressively up the esophagus. The absence of esophagitis above a stricture sug-

5

gests a drug-induced injury or a neoplasm, which should always be ruled out by tissue biopsy.

Because columnar epithelium is more resistant to acid,[11] Barrett's esophagus is associated with the alleviation of heartburn. According to a study of patients known to have the esophageal changes of Barrett's, 25% had no symptoms of reflux.[12] It is not uncommon for such patients to remain asymptomatic for many years until the development of an associated complication.[3]

Two recent studies have addressed the acid versus alkaline reflux question in the causation of Barrett's esophagus. Kauer and associates demonstrated that reflux of bilirubin occurs in Barrett's patients significantly more than in normal volunteers, raising the possibility that esophageal injury may occur at high pH levels.[13] However, Vaezi and colleagues reported data showing that an acidic pH is required for bile acids to damage esophageal mucosa.[14]

Another study presents clinical evidence that complications associated with the Barrett's changes are secondary to refluxed alkalinized duodenogastric juice.[15] According to Attwood and colleagues, patients with Barrett's esophagus were subject to greater alkaline as well as acid exposure than those with esophagitis.[15] Furthermore, alkaline exposure was greater in patients with complications of Barrett's (stricture, ulceration, carcinoma) than in those without.

Given these somewhat confusing findings, it seems likely that alkaline reflux and other noxious agents play some role in the development of Barrett's esophagus, with acid damage remaining the primary pathogenic mechanism.

The development of Barrett's epithelium remains the most disconcerting complication of reflux disease because of its predisposition to carcinoma.[16] Two recent studies suggest the incidence of adenocarcinoma is one in 96 to 99 patient-years in follow-up.[17,18]

According to recent evidence, adenocarcinoma in Barrett's epithelium occurs only in conjunction with or following the development of dysplastic changes.[17-19] The value of endoscopic surveillance in patients with Barrett's epithelium no longer is controversial. Although optimal frequency of endoscopic follow-up is not yet known, recent data suggest the following guidelines:[16]

- A routine surveillance program is mandatory, with biopsies in a defined pattern covering four quadrants every 2 cm.
- In patients with no dysplasia, surveillance intervals can probably be longer than 1 year.
- If high-grade dysplasia is found and confirmed, resection is appropriate for good surgical candidates; frequent surveillance (at least semiannually) remains a less desirable alternative.

REFERENCES

1. Peters JH, DeMeester TR. Gastroesophageal reflux. *Surg Clin North Am*. 1993;73:1119-1144.

2. Jessurun J, Yardley JH, Giardiello FM, Hamilton SR. Intracytoplasmic plasma proteins in distended esophageal squamous cells (balloon cells). *Mod Pathol.* 1988;1:175-181.

3. Morton LS, Fromkes JJ. Gastroesophageal reflux disease: diagnosis and medical therapy. *Geriatrics*. 1993;48:60-66.

4. Ippoliti A. Inflammatory and infectious esophageal disorders. In: Gitnick G, ed. *Principles and Practice of Gastroenterology and Hepatology*, 2nd ed. Norwalk, Conn: Appleton & Lange; 1994:37-49.

5. Bozymski EM. Pathophysiology and diagnosis of gastroesophageal reflux disease. *Am J Hosp Pharm*. 1993;50 (suppl 1):S4-S6.

6. Palmer ED. The hiatus hernia–esophagitis–esophageal stricture complex: twenty-year prospective study. *Am J Med.* 1968;44:566-579.

7. Bonavina L, DeMeester TR, McChesney L, Schwizer W, Albertucci M, Bailey RT. Drug-induced esophageal strictures. *Ann Surg.* 1987;206:173-183.

8. Cameron AJ, Zinsmeister DR, Ballard AJ, Carney JA. Prevalence of columnar-lined (Barrett's) esophagus. Comparison of population-based clinical and autopsy findings. *Gastroenterology.* 1990;99:918-922.

9. Green PHR. What is the prevalence of Barrett's in the general population and in patients with GERD? Syllabus, NY Soc Gastrointest Endosc Postgrad Course. November 10-11, 1994:2-3

10. Zeroogian JM, Spechler SJ, Antonioli DA, Wang HH, Goyal RK. The high prevalence of short-segment Barrett's esophagus. *Gastroenterology.* 1994;106:A216. Abstract.

11. Johnson DA, Winters C, Spurling TJ, Chobanian SJ, Cattau EL Jr. Esophageal acid sensitivity in Barrett's esophagus. *J Clin Gastroenterol.* 1987;9:23-27.

12. Spechler SJ. Barrett's esophagus: what's new and what to do. *Am J Gastroenterol.* 1989;84:220-223. Editorial.

13. Kauer WK, Ireland AP, Burdiles P, Clark GWB, Peters JH, DeMeester TR. The correlation between bile and acid reflux in Barrett's esophagus. *Gastroenterology.* 1994; 106:A104. Abstract.

14. Vaezi MF, Champion GL, Richter JE. Role of duodenogastroesophageal reflux (DGER) and bile acids in the development of Barrett's esophagus. *Gastroenterology.* 1994;106:A201. Abstract.

15. Attwood SE, DeMeester TR, Bremner CG, Barlow AP, Hinder RA. Alkaline gastroesophageal reflux: implications in the development of complications in Barrett's columnar-lined lower esophagus. *Surgery.* 1989;106:764-770.

16. Clouse RE, Chokshi HR. The esophagus. In: Gitnick G, ed. *Current Gastroenterology*, Volume 14. St. Louis, Mo: Mosby–Year Book, Inc; 1994:1-28.

17. Williamson WA, Ellis FH Jr, Gibb SP, et al. Barrett's esophagus: prevalence and incidence of adenocarcinoma. *Arch Intern Med*. 1991;151:2212-2216.

18. Miros M, Kerlin P, Walker N. Only patients with dysplasia progress to adenocarcinoma in Barrett's oesophagus. *Gut*. 1991;32:1441-1446.

19. Reid BJ, Blount PL, Rubin CE, Levine DS, Haggitt RC, Rabinovitch PS. Flow-cytometric and histological progression to malignancy in Barrett's esophagus: prospective endoscopic surveillance of a cohort. *Gastroenterology*. 1992;102:1212-1219.

PART 3

THERAPY FOR GASTROESOPHAGEAL REFLUX DISEASE

6 Nonpharmacologic Management

The primary goal of gastrointestinal esophageal reflux disease (GERD) therapy is complete resolution of symptoms arising from esophageal mucosal contact with refluxed acidic gastric content,[1] which often means minimizing or eliminating reflux.[1] Concomitant therapeutic endpoints include:

- Healing esophagitis when present
- Prevention of complications
- Maintenance of remission.

In many, indeed most GERD patients, symptomatic resolution is a major aim. In those with esophagitis, however, relief without healing results in a continuing cycle of destruction—reflux, esophageal inflammation, compromised lower esophageal sphincter (LES), reflux.[2] The result, increasingly severe esophagitis, carries a risk of complications such as peptic stricture or Barrett's esophagus.[3] Risk factors associated with these complications are not well identified, nor is there any direct evidence that healing of esophagitis will prevent their development. The possibility is supported, however, by many anecdotes regarding the resolution of peptic stricture by antireflux surgery. Theoretically, therefore, maintained healing will prevent the development or progression of Barrett's esophagus.

Therapeutic intervention can be divided into three phases (Table 6.1):

- Lifestyle changes
- Pharmacologic manipulation of acid secretion, concentration and transport
- Surgery.

TABLE 6.1 — MANAGEMENT PHASES IN THE TREATMENT OF GERD

Phase 1
- Modify diet if symptoms are related to diet
- Lose weight if overweight (is always beneficial)
- Reduce smoking and alcohol intake (is always beneficial)
- Elevate head of bed if nocturnal symptoms or severe esophagitis are present
- Avoid certain drugs if they are related to symptoms

Phase 2
- Antacids
- Alginic acid
- Sucralfate
- Prokinetic drugs
- H_2-receptor antagonists
- Acid pump inhibitors

Phase 3
- Antireflux surgery

Modified from: Garnett WR. Efficacy, safety and cost issues in managing patients with gastroesophageal reflux disease. *Am J Hosp Pharm.* 1993;50(suppl 1):S11-S18.

Lifestyle Changes

There is a consensus that all patients with reflux symptoms should make lifestyle adjustments as a first step if lifestyle seems related to symptoms (Table 6.1).[2] Indeed, very simple measures can lead to marked reductions of reflux symptoms in patients whose symptoms seem obviously linked to lifestyle[2] and perhaps in some with moderate symptoms. Such adjustments alone should not be expected to provide significant relief in most patients, however.

■ Avoid Supine Position After Meals

As has been noted, reflux is more frequent after meals and during periods of increased intra-abdominal pressure. Furthermore, esophageal clearance may be markedly delayed when the body is supine, and particularly during sleep when salivation and swallowing are minimal.[1,4] It follows, therefore, that patients should:

- Not lie down soon after eating
- Not eat for two to three hours before bedtime

■ Dietary Restriction

Gastric volume can be reduced by avoiding large meals and bedtime snacks.[1] Although the significance of meal size and types of food eaten has received little attention in formal studies, experience shows that these variables influence the severity of postprandial reflux symptoms.[3]

The association of meal size with reflux-induced heartburn and nonspecific dyspepsia, though reasonable, seems to have fostered the idea that GERD is a disease of overindulgence rather than of disordered physiology.[3] This viewpoint ignores the fact that in many patients, symptoms occur after only modest food intake.

Gastric distention is a well-defined provocative factor for reflux,[5] but it is unclear how certain foods provoke heartburn; some may trigger reflux directly, others may irritate the gastric mucosa. In fact, the value of dietary restriction is more folklore than science.[4] The ingestion of certain foods, such as fats, peppermint, and chocolate, has been shown to decrease LES resting pressure, but no association has been found between specific food and reflux or heartburn. Strict adherence to a bland diet or frequent small meals is not necessary for the treatment of GERD. Rather simple avoidance of foods that provoke symptoms is sufficient.

In short, dietary modifications should perhaps be suggested, but with the knowledge that they are often ineffective as well as difficult for some patients to maintain.[3]

■ Obesity

Obesity is considered by many to be an important determinant of LES incompetence, giving further support to the association of GERD with overindulgence.[3] The traditional and relatively untested view that obesity puts stress on the antireflux mechanism has not been supported by recent studies. Furthermore, there is no convincing evidence that reflux disease is particularly common in obese patients or that weight loss reduces symptoms.

■ Smoking

Another "indulgence," smoking, also has been thought to play a major role in the production of GERD.[3] Now it seems cessation of smoking is not, perhaps, as critical as previously suggested.[6] Cigarette smoking probably exacerbates GERD by the direct provocation of acid reflux and, perhaps, by a long-lasting reduction of LES pressure.[7] Cigarette smoking has also been implicated in the severity and healing rate of esophagitis.[8] However, there are no convincing data to indicate that cessation of smoking achieves effective relief of reflux-induced symptoms.[3]

■ Alcohol

Alcohol diminishes the amplitude of the LES, peristaltic supine waves, and frequency of contraction.[9,10] Prolonged supine reflux does occur particularly when alcohol is ingested shortly before bedtime.[11] Nevertheless, alcohol does not seem to be an independent determining factor in GERD.[3]

■ Elevating the Head of the Bed

Elevating the head of the bed by six inches will improve esophageal clearance and protect the esophagus during sleep when swallowing and salivation are minimal.[1] This position cannot be achieved merely by sleeping on several pillows.[4] Some patients have found a foam wedge to be an effective and more comfortable way to raise the upper body (Figure 6.1).[12]

However, the majority of GERD patients should not be instructed to undertake this measure. Given the modest benefit to be gained by such elevation,[3,12,13] and that some patients find it intolerable, it should be restricted to those with nocturnal symptoms or severe disease. According to pH monitoring studies, in the majority of patients, most acid exposure occurs during the day after meals.[14]

■ Drugs

Certain medications may lower LES pressure. Several others may cause direct mucosal damage as a result of a tablet or capsule's prolonged contact with the esophageal epithelium and slow clearance into the stomach.[15] Patients should be instructed to sit or stand and drink plenty of water when taking such drugs and to avoid taking them at bedtime.

Several studies suggest that nonsteroidal anti-inflammatory drugs (NSAIDs) are associated with esophageal damage, especially in patients with GERD.[16-19] In two of these studies, NSAIDs were linked to the development of esophageal strictures.[17,18] Another found a previously unreported strong association of aspirin use with esophagitis, suggesting that aspirin may play a significant role in the resistance of esophagitis to therapy, as well as relapse after a short-term course is completed.[19]

FIGURE 6.1—IMPACT OF BEDHEAD ELEVATION ON NIGHT-TIME ESOPHAGEAL ACID EXPOSURE

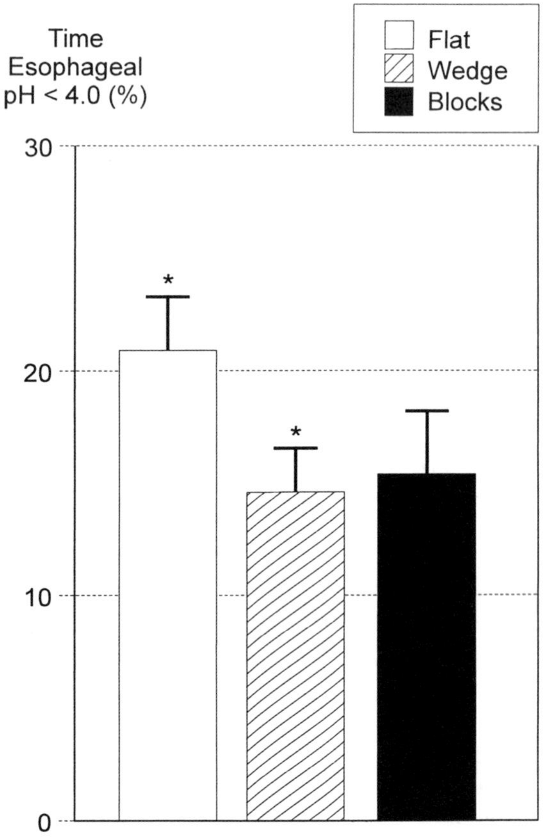

* $P < 0.05$.

Impact of 19-cm bedhead elevation (blocks) or a foam wedge pillow on night-time esophageal acid exposure.

Hamilton JW, Boisen RJ, Yamamoto DT, Wagner JL, Reichelderfer M. Sleeping on a wedge diminishes exposure of the esophagus to refluxed acid. *Dig Dis Sci*. 1988;33: 518-522. Reprinted with permission.

REFERENCES

1. Morton LS, Fromkes JJ. Gastroesophageal reflux disease: diagnosis and medical therapy. *Geriatrics*. 1993;48:60-66.

2. Garnett WR. Efficacy, safety and cost issues in managing patients with gastroesophageal reflux disease. *Am J Hosp Pharm*. 1993;50(suppl 1):S11-S18.

3. Dent J. Long-term aims of treatment of reflux disease, and the role of non-drug measures. *Digestion*. 1992;51 (suppl 1):30-34.

4. Ippoliti A. Inflammatory and infectious esophageal disorders. In: Gitnick G, ed. *Principles and Practice of Gastroenterology and Hepatology*, 2nd ed. Norwalk, Conn: Appleton & Lange; 1994:37-49.

5. Holloway RH, Hongo M, Berger K, McCallum RW. Gastric distension: a mechanism for postprandial gastroesophageal reflux. *Gastroenterology*. 1985;89:779-784.

6. Waring JP, Eastwood TF, Austin JM, Sanowski RA. The immediate effects of cessation of cigarette smoking on gastroesophageal reflux. *Am Gastroenterol*. 1989;84: 1076-1078.

7. Kahrilas PJ, Gupta RR. Mechanisms of acid reflux associated with cigarette smoking. *Gut*. 1990;31:4-10.

8. Koelz HR, Birchler R, Bretholz A, et al. Healing and relapse of reflux esophagitis during treatment with ranitidine. *Gastroenterology*. 1986;91:1198-1205.

9. Hogan WJ, Viegas de Andrade SR, Winship DH. Ethanol-induced acute esophageal motor dysfunction. *J Appl Physiol*. 1972;32:755-760.

10. Mayer EN, Grabowski CJ, Fisher RS. Effects of graded doses of alcohol upon esophageal motor function. *Gastroenterology*. 1978;75;1133-1136.

11. Vitale GC, Cheadle WG, Patel B, Sadek SA, Michel ME, Cuschieri A. The effect of alcohol on nocturnal gastroesophageal reflux. *JAMA*. 1987;258:2077-2079.

12. Hamilton JW, Boisen RJ, Yamamoto DT, Wagner JL, Reichelderfer M. Sleeping on a wedge diminishes exposure of the esophagus to refluxed acid. *Dig Dis Sci*. 1988; 33:518-522.

13. Johnson LF, DeMeester TR. Evaluation of elevation of the head of the bed, bethanechol, and antacid foam tablets on gastroesophageal reflux. *Dig Dis Sci*. 1981;26: 673-680.

14. de Caestecker JS, Blackwell JN, Pryde A, Heading RC. Daytime gastro-oesophageal reflux is important in oesophagitis. *Gut*. 1987;28:519-526.

15. Porro GB, Pace F. Rationale and efficacy of medical therapy for gastro-oesophageal reflux disease. *J Intern Med*. 1993;234:387-396.

16. Sontag S, Schnel T, Mak E, et al. NSAIDS with or without prednisone: bad news for the gut mucosa. *Gastroenterology*. 1989;96:A483. Abstract.

17. Heller SR, Fellows IW, Ogilvie AL, Atkinson M. Non-steroidal anti-inflammatory drugs and benign oesophageal stricture. *Br Med J*. 1982;285:167-168.

18. Wilkins WE, Ridley MG, Pozniak AL. Benign stricture of the oesophagus: role of non-steroidal anti-inflammatory drugs. *Gut*. 1984;25:478-480.

19. Lanas A, Hirschowitz BI. Significant role of aspirin use in patients with esophagitis. *J Clin Gastroenterol*. 1991; 13:622-627.

7 Pharmacologic Management

The place of traditional nondrug measures in gastroesophageal reflux disease (GERD) is being redefined by the high efficacy and low morbidity of acid-inhibitory therapy,[1] predominantly the antisecretory agents (Table 7.1).[2] The rationale for the use of these and other agents used in the treatment of GERD is best understood in terms of the physiologic regulation of acid secretion.

The stomach is lined by a columnar epithelium of surface mucous cells that extend into gastric pits containing the secretory glands.[3] The oxyntic glands of the gastric fundus and body are composed primarily of acid-forming parietal cells and chief, or peptic cells, that secrete pepsinogen. Substances that affect parietal cell secretion are released by a number of endocrine-paracrine cells (histamine, somatostatin, serotonin, and other peptide hormones) at the base of the gastric glands, and by G cells of the pyloric, or antral glands. Acetylcholine, histamine and gastrin all stimulate the parietal cell directly to secrete HCl.[4] Pepsin, the active form of pepsinogen, is a proteolytic enzyme that begins the process of protein digestion.[4]

Along the parietal cell's membrane are three classes of receptors:

- Histamine—paracrine receptors
- Gastrin—endocrine receptors
- Acetylcholine—neurocrine (muscarinic) receptors.

All mediate the final step in the secretion of hydrochloric acid, activation of the H^+/K^+-ATPase acid pump.[3]

TABLE 7.1 —COMPARISON OF AGENTS AVAILABLE FOR TREATING GERD

Agent(s)	Relief of Symptoms	Promotion of Healing	Adverse Effects	Drug Interactions	Frequency of Administration	Patient Acceptance
Antacids, alginic acid	Fair	Poor	Many	Many	Frequent	Fair
H_2-Receptor antagonists	Good	Fair	Some*	Some*	bid†	Good
Sucralfate	Fair	Poor	Few	Few	qid‡	Fair
Prokinetic agents	Fair	Poor	Many	Few	qid	Poor
Acid pump inhibitors	Excellent	Good	Few	Few	Once daily	Excellent

* Especially with cimetidine † Large doses may be necessary ‡ Must be given in liquid form to relieve symptoms

Modified from: Garnett WR. Efficacy, safety and cost issues in managing patients with gastroesophageal reflux disease. *Am J Hosp Pharm*. 1993;50(suppl 1):S11-S18.

Gastric acid secretion in response to a mixed meal (protein, carbohydrate, and fat) occurs in three phases (Table 7.2):[3]

- The cephalic phase is initiated by the thought, smell, sight, and taste of food. This phase stimulates afferent, neural signals to the brainstem and, in turn, vagal efferent fibers to parietal and antral gland regions of the stomach.
- The more prolonged gastric phase is mediated by gastric distention—which activates both long, vagovagal reflexes and short, intragastric cholinergic reflexes—and by chemical reactions of food with the gastric mucosa[5] (Figure 7.1).
- The intestinal phase occurs after the stomach empties into the duodenum, and is probably stimulated by the absorption of intestinal amino acids and their entry into the circulation.[3] Total duration of the postprandial secretory response is about four hours.

Basal or interdigestive secretion occurs in the absence of environmental and gastrointestinal stimulation.[3] Basal secretion adheres to a circadian rhythm. Secretion is lowest between 5 AM and 11 AM, and highest in the evening between approximately 7 PM and 1 AM.

Of the currently available agents used to treat the symptoms of GERD, antacids, the traditional mainstay of medical therapy for heartburn, neutralize gastric acid and, as a result of gastric alkalinization, increase LES pressure.[6] The antacids have no direct influence on gastric acid secretion, and because their effect is so short-lived, they are not considered primary agents for the treatment of GERD.[2] The specifically antireflux agents available in the United States are listed in Table 7.3.

Both the H_2-receptor antagonists (H_2-RAs) and the acid pump inhibitors (APIs) block acid secretion: H_2-RAs block histamine receptors on the parietal cell

7

TABLE 7.2 — PHASES/INITIATORS/PATHS TO AND MEDIATORS AT THE PARIETAL CELL

Phase	Initiator	Path	Mediator
Cephalic	Feeding, sham or real*	Direct vagal Vagal-antral gastrin-blood	Acetylcholine Gastrin
	Impairment of supply utilization of glucose by brain		
Gastric	Distention*	Vagovagal reflexes (same two postganglionic paths as for cephalic phase) Local intramural reflexes (same two postganglionic paths as for cephalic phase)	Acetylcholine Gastrin
	Calcium, amino acids, peptides	Release of gastrin into blood by intraluminal action on G cells	Gastrin
Intestinal	Distension	At least in part by release into blood unidentified hormone	Enterooxyntin (postulated)
	Amino acids and peptides	At least in part by amino acids absorbed into blood	Amino acids

* In mechanisms involving both direct neural action on the parietal cell and neural release of gastrin, the relative importance of these two components varies with species, initiators, and conditions of testing.

Debas HT. Peripheral regulation of gastric acid secretion. In: Johnson LR, Christensen J, Jackson MJ, Jacobson ED, Walsh JH, eds. *Physiology of the Gastrointestinal Tract*, 2nd ed., vol. 2. New York, NY: Raven Press; 1987:933. Reprinted with permission.

FIGURE 7.1—STIMULATION OF THE PARIETAL CELL

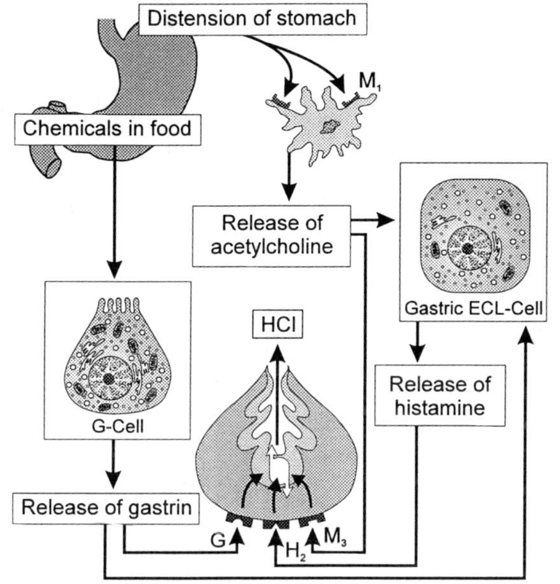

The digestive (gastric) phase of acid secretion by the parietal cell is mediated by distention of the stomach, which activates vagovagal and cholinergic reflexes, and by reactions of the chemicals in food with the gastric mucosa. Acetylcholine, released from enteric nerve fibers in the fundic mucosa, stimulates the secretion of HCl directly by binding to its receptor on the parietal cell and indirectly via stimulation of gastric ECL (enterochromaffin-like) cells to release histamine. Gastrin, released by the antral G cells in response to polypeptides and amino-acids in the stomach contents, also provides both direct and indirect stimulation of parietal cell activation.

M_1=muscarinic (neurocrine) receptor for acetylcholine; M_3=muscarinic receptor; G=gastrin (endocrine) receptor; H_2=histamine (paracrine) receptor.

Adapted from: Sachs G, Hersey SJ. *The Gastric Parietal Cell*. Oxford, UK: Oxford Clinical Communications; 1994:26. Reprinted with permission.

7

TABLE 7.3 — ANTIREFLUX MEDICATIONS USED IN THE TREATMENT OF GERD IN THE UNITED STATES

Agent: Generic (Trade) Name	Indication	Recommended Dosage
H_2-Receptor Antagonists		
Cimetidine (Tagamet)	GERD	1600 mg/d in divided doses (800 mg bid or 400 mg qid) for 12 weeks
Famotidine (Pepcid)	GERD	20 mg bid for up to 6 weeks
	Erosive esophagitis	20 or 40 mg bid for up to 12 weeks
Nizatidine (Axid Pulvules)	Erosive esophagitis/heartburn due to GERD	150 mg bid for up to 12 weeks
Ranitidine (Zantac)	GERD	150 mg or 10 mL (2 teaspoons equivalent to 150 mg of ranitidine) bid
	Erosive esophagitis	150 mg or 10 mL (2 teaspoons equivalent to 150 mg of ranitidine) qid
	Maintenance of healing of erosive esophagitis	150 mg or 10 mL (2 teaspoons equivalent to 150 mg of ranitidine) bid

Prokinetic Drugs		
Cisapride (Propulsid)	Symptomatic treatment of nocturnal heartburn due to GERD	10-20 mg qid at least 15 minutes before meals and at bedtime
Metoclopramide (Reglan)	Symptomatic gastroesophageal reflux	10-15 mg up to qid, 30 minutes before each meal and at bedtime for 4-12 weeks
H^+/K^+-ATPase (acid pump) Inhibitors		
Lansoprazole (Prevacid)	Erosive esophagitis	30 mg/d for up to 8 weeks
	Maintenance of healing of erosive esophagitis	15 mg/d
Omeprazole (Prilosec)	Erosive esophagitis or poorly responsive symptomatic GERD	20 mg/d for 4-8 weeks
	Maintenance of healing of erosive esophagitis	20 mg/d

Physicians' Desk Reference®, 51st ed. Montvale, NJ: Medical Economics Data Production Company; 1997:516-519, 1182-1184, 1346-1348, 1468-1470, 1763-1765, 2243-2245, 2694-2697, 2746-2748.

surface;[2,7] the APIs act within the parietal cell to block the gastric acid pump, the final mediator of acid secretion.[2] Sucralfate has no effect on acid secretion, rather it may form a barrier to prevent penetration of acid into the gastrointestinal mucosa.[2] The prokinetic agents may increase LES tone, esophageal clearance, and gastric emptying in some patients.

Antacids

All antacids—sodium bicarbonate, calcium carbonate, aluminum and magnesium hydroxide—work by neutralizing the gastric acid secreted by parietal cells, thus increasing the intragastric pH. A pH above 4.0 results in at least a 95% reduction in the formation of pepsin and the resulting acid-pepsin complex. The neutralizing effects of antacids differ from patient to patient, however, and optimum dosages are not known. Two reports suggest that antacids also may increase the LES pressure, thus decreasing reflux.[6]

Adverse effects of antacids include:[2]

- The potential for altering systemic pH (sodium bicarbonate)
- Stimulation of acid production through release of gastrin (calcium carbonate)
- Hypercalcemia (calcium carbonate)
- Constipation (aluminum hydroxide)
- Diarrhea (magnesium hydroxide).

Antacids have a short duration of action: 45 to 60 minutes during fasting, 1 to 3 hours if administered 1 hour after meals.[2] Because they may interact with other drugs by altering the rate or extent of absorption as well as renal elimination of some agents, antacids should be taken at least 2 hours before or after other medications.

Antacids provide symptomatic relief in many patients with mild to moderate GERD, particularly those whose symptoms occur less frequently than daily.[8] Most patients with chronic symptoms have already failed on antacids when they are first seen by a physician. There are no data to indicate antacids promote healing of eroded esophageal mucosa.[2,9]

Alginic Acid

Although alginic acid preparations contain small quantities of antacid, they do not alter intragastric pH.[2] Rather, the antacid converts alginic acid to sodium alginate, which floats on top of the gastric contents, thus providing a nonerosive reflux. The agent is well tolerated, at least as effective as antacids in the relief of symptoms of mild to moderate GERD, and can be administered less often than antacids. It has not been shown to promote the healing of eroded esophageal mucosa.

Histamine$_2$-Receptor Antagonists

The four currently available H_2-RAs are:[2]

- Cimetidine
- Famotidine
- Nizatidine
- Ranitidine.

All act competitively and reversibly to inhibit stimulation of the parietal cell by histamine.[10] The degree of inhibition parallels the concentration of the drug in plasma over a wide range.

The H_2-RAs also inhibit acid secretion elicited by gastrin. An important advantage of these agents is their inhibition of basal and nocturnal acid secretion. In addition, they reduce both the volume of gastric juice secreted and its hydrogen ion concentration, resulting in a parallel fall in pepsin output. The H_2-RAs have no consistent effect on the rate of gastric emptying, LES pressure, or pancreatic secretion.[10]

Bioavailability of the H_2-RAs ranges from 50% to 90%.[2] Approximately 70% of a dose is excreted unchanged in the urine, with the other 30% undergoing oxidation in the liver.

The H_2-RAs differ in strength, with cimetidine the least and famotidine the most potent. Standard doses of H_2-RAs will usually alleviate symptoms of GERD and may heal mild-to-moderate esophagitis.[11] High-dose (twofold or more standard dose) may also heal high-grade lesions, but the reported experience is small.[12]

For example, healing frequencies with cimetidine, 800 mg/day to 1600 mg/day for 6 weeks, are typically 60% to 70% in grade 1 or minimal esophagitis, but drop to 20% to 30% for grade 3, circumferential erosions.[12] When treatment is extended for 12 weeks, healing frequencies increase from 80% to 90% and 40% to 50%, respectively, in most studies.

Controlled trials comparing "standard dose" regimens of cimetidine and the lower dose ranitidine (150 mg bid) to not demonstrate significant differences in therapeutic outcome.[12]

■ Maintenance Therapy

In two multicenter, double-blind, randomized, placebo-controlled, 48-week trials conducted in patients whose erosive esophagitis had been previously healed, ranitidine 150 mg bid was significantly more effective than placebo in maintaining healing of erosive esophagitis.[12] The recommended adult oral dosage of ranitadine for the maintenance of healing of erosive esophagitis is 150 mg twice daily. Placebo-controlled trials have been carried out for 48 weeks.

Although the H_2-RAs are remarkably safe drugs, adverse effects can occur, such as:

- Central nervous system (CNS) effects (cimetidine, in high concentrations)[2]
- Headache
- Diarrhea
- Gynecomastia and impotence (cimetidine, in prolonged use of large doses).[7]

Sucralfate

An aluminum complex of a polysulfate sucrose molecule, sucralfate disassociates in the acidic medium of the stomach and forms polyvalent bonds with both normal and eroded mucosa.[2] It binds bile acids and pepsin, and stimulates the synthesis and release of gastric mucosal prostaglandins as well as bicarbonate and the epidermal growth factor that stimulates healing.[14]

Sucralfate's pharmacologic effect is entirely local. Its primary adverse effect is constipation. Because aluminum is released when sucralfate dissociates, chelates may be formed if it is administered simultaneously with other drugs.[15]

Although studies of the drug's effectiveness in healing esophageal erosions are limited, indications are that sucralfate may be comparable to standard dosages of the H_2-RAs cimetidine[16] and ranitidine[17] in promoting healing.

Prokinetic Drugs

7

Can the motility defect in GERD be favorably influenced by a pharmacologic approach?[13] A recent detailed review of the effects of promotility drugs on GERD concludes that physiologic promise may not predict clinical success.[13] The clinical efficacy of the early agents—metoclopramide, bethanechol, domperidone—was never consistently confirmed.[19] This was true for a number of reasons:[19]

- Although they may increase LES pressure, these drugs have minimal effect when basal LES is low
- No evidence of any effect on transient LES relaxations (TLESRs)
- An inconsistent effect on esophageal peristalsis
- Can enhance gastric emptying acutely, not on long-term administration
- Not predictably effective in healing
- Clinical use limited because of side effects.

The most recently approved agent cisapride may, however, play a role in the treatment of GERD.[19] In European studies, cisapride was shown to be effective in enhancing LES pressure and esophageal peristalsis as well as accelerating gastric emptying. Furthermore, the drug effectively relieved GERD symptoms and healed grades I to II esophagitis with minimal side effects or tachyphylaxis.

Although US studies support the efficacy of cisapride for the relief of nocturnal heartburn, they have not found such high healing rates.[19] Moreover, it is not yet clear whether the agent is effective in erosive esophagitis.

Two studies have evaluated the efficacy of combination therapy with cisapride and an H_2-RA, one with cimetidine,[15] the other with ranitidine.[21] The cimetidine/cisapride combination relieved diurnal and nocturnal heartburn (in 6 to 12 weeks) more effectively than cimetidine alone.[20] In the ranitidine/cisapride trial, no significant difference in healing was seen between the combination and ranitidine alone at 6 weeks.[21]

Among patients remaining in the ranitidine/cisapride study for 12 weeks, the number with severe esophagitis was reduced by half in the combination group, but was unchanged in those receiving ranitidine alone. However, because of the small number of patients, this difference was not significant.

The Acid Pump Inhibitors

The secretion of hydrochloric acid by gastric parietal cells ultimately depends on the function of the acid (hydrogen ion) pump.[10] This pump is H^+/K^+-ATPase, an enzyme that uses the energy released by the metabolism of ATP to move protons (actually, hydronium ions) across parietal cell membranes in exchange for potassium ions.[22]

In the nonsecretory state, H^+/K^+-ATPase is situated in tubulovesicles in the parietal cell cytoplasm.[22] Since the vesicles contain no potassium and the vesicular membranes are impermeable to potassium ions, the pump is inactive.

On activation of the parietal cell, by histamine for example, the tubulovesicles transform into secretory canaliculi,[23] with the enzyme translocated to their permeable plasma membranes.[22] The H^+/K^+-ATPase is now exposed to potassium ions and, in the presence of the canaliculi's membrane permeability, can now secrete acid at a pH of about 1.0.

The acid pump inhibitors are weak bases that are absorbed in the intestine and reach the parietal cell through the bloodstream.[22] At a pH of about 7.0, the drugs are not charged and can cross cell membranes. However, once in the secretory canaliculi of actively-secreting cells, the inhibitory agents are exposed to a pH of less than 2.0. Thus, they are protonated at different rates to the active drug, which provides prolonged inhibition of H^+/K^+-ATPase and, in turn, of acid secretion, regardless of the stimulus (Figure 7.2).[24]

The acid pump inhibitors approach the perfect therapeutic profile in terms of degree and duration of acid suppression.[24]

For both the available agents, lansoprazole and omeprazole, timing of administration is an important factor, however.[24] For example, lansoprazole, 30 mg

FIGURE 7.2 — ACTION OF ANTISECRETORY AGENTS ON THE GASTRIC PARIETAL CELL

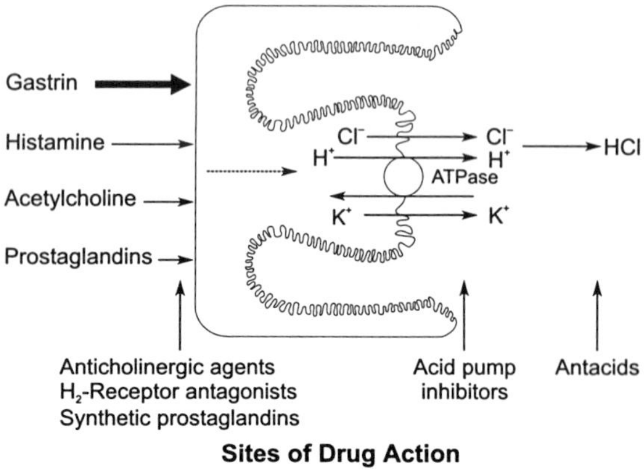

When the parietal cell is activated, H^+/K^+-ATPase (the acid pump) is translocated from tubulovesicles in the cytoplasm to the permeable membranes of secretory canaliculi, where it mediates the secretion of gastric acid. The acid pump inhibitors block the final common pathway of acid secretion on the apical region of the cell, whereas histamine H_2-receptor antagonists and anticholinergic agents block receptors on its basolateral surface.

Spencer CM, Faulds D. Lansoprazole. A reappraisal of its pharmacodynamic and pharmacokinetic properties, and its therapeutic efficacy in acid-related disorders. *Drugs*. 1994;48:404. Reprinted with permission.

given once a day, provides a significantly greater decrease in 24-hour intragastric acidity when administered at 8 AM than at 10 PM.[24] Similar differences in duration of acid suppression were seen with omeprazole, 20 mg given morning and night.

■ **Safety**

The development of these increasingly potent and long-acting inhibitors of acid secretion raised fears that profound inhibition of acid secretion may be unsafe.[25] Studies have shown that the alterations in gastric mucosal morphology observed in rats administered very high doses of omeprazole for prolonged periods represent the effects of hypergastrinemia occurring in response to profound inhibition of acid secretion.[26] Also, during the lifetime exposure of rats with up to 150 mg/kg/day of lansoprazole dosed 7 days a week, marked hypergastrinemia was observed, followed by ECL cell proliferation and formation of carcinoid tumors.[27]

Proliferation of enterochromaffin-like (ECL) cells in the oxyntic mucosa and the development of ECL-cell carcinoids has also been observed in rats with other antisecretory agents (including ranitidine) and following partial corpectomy.[26]

However, gastric biopsy specimens from the body of the stomach from approximately 150 patients treated continuously with lansoprazole for at least 1 year have not shown evidence of ECL cell effects similar to those seen in rat studies.[27] For example, in a 4-year study of lansoprazole, 30 mg/day to 60 mg/day, no dysplasia of ECL cells was observed in 40 patients with acid-related disorders, although the volume density of argyrophilic cells in the oxyntic mucosa increased slightly.[28]

In another study, ECL cell hyperplasia developed in some patients with refractory peptic ulcers or reflux esophagitis who received lansoprazole, 30 mg/day to 120 mg/day for 30 months. Mean basal gastrin levels increased after 3 months of treatment and then plateaued. ECL cell density increased continuously from baseline but was not correlated with serum gastrin levels. No dysplastic lesions or carcinoids were noted in any patients.

Variable degrees of mucosal cell hyperplasia and gastric atrophy have been reported to develop in some patients receiving long-term therapy with omeprazole, however, no reports have been published showing gastric atrophy in those receiving lansoprazole.[28]

Although lansoprazole is metabolized through the cytochrome P_{450} system, studies have shown that it does not have clinically significant interactions with other agents metabolized by that system, such as warfarin, antipyrine, indomethacin, ibuprofen, phenytoin, propranolol, prednisone, or diazepam in healthy subjects.[27] When lansoprazole was administered concomitantly with theophylline, a minor increase (10%) in the clearance of theophylline was seen. Although unlikely to be of clinical concern, individual patients may require additional titration of theophylline dosage when lansoprazole is started or stopped to ensure clinically effective blood levels.

Finally, coadministration of lansoprazole with sucralfate delayed absorption and reduced lansoprazole bioavailability by approximately 30%. Thus, lansoprazole should be taken at least 30 minutes before sucralfate.

Omeprazole can prolong the elimination of diazepam, warfarin, and phenytoin, and there have been reports of interaction with other drugs metabolized by the cytochrome P_{450} system, such as cyclosporine, disulfiram, and benzodiazepines.[29] Patients should be monitored to determine whether it is necessary to adjust the dosage of these drugs when taken concomitantly with omeprazole. In normal subjects, no interaction with theophylline or propranolol was found.

Theoretically, because of their profound and long-lasting inhibition of gastric acid secretion, both lansoprazole and omeprazole may interfere with the absorption of drugs where gastric pH is an important determinant of bioavailability, eg, ketoconazole, ampicillin esters, iron salts, and digoxin.[27,29]

Concomitant administration of either lansoprazole or omeprazole with antacids in clinical trials did not interfere with the effects of either.

■ Recommended Dosages

The acid pump inhibitors are the only drugs in the GERD armamentarium that are recommended to be taken once a day, thus promoting compliance.[30]

Lansoprazole

A short-term (up to 8 weeks) course of lansoprazole, 30 mg/day, is indicated for healing and symptom relief in patients:[27]

- With all grades of erosive esophagitis
- Who do not heal on lansoprazole 8-week course
- Who experience a recurrence of erosive esophagitis.

Lansoprazole is also indicated for maintenance of healing of erosive esophagitis at a dose of 15 mg once daily.

Omeprazole

Similar short-term (4 to 8 weeks) courses of omeprazole, 20 mg/day, are indicated for patients:[29]

- With erosive esophagitis diagnosed by endoscopy
- With GERD poorly responsive to customary medical treatment
- With recurrence of erosive esophagitis or poorly responsive GERD
- With GERD unresponsive to the initial 8-week course.

For maintenance of healing of erosive esophagitis, the adult dose of omeprazole is 20 mg/day.

■ **Efficacy**

Acid pump inhibitors are clearly the most effective available medical therapy for reflux disease.[31] Patients who have no endoscopic abnormalities or who have minor erosive esophagitis may do well on an H_2-RA. For those who fail to respond, however, an API should be considered.

In randomized, controlled trials, lansoprazole has yielded both significantly greater healing rates and significantly better symptomatic relief than ranitidine.[32-34] And in recent, randomized, multicenter, double-blind trials, lansoprazole provided similar healing and greater early symptom relief than omeprazole (Table 7.4).[34,35]

For patients presenting for the first time with more extensive erosive or ulcerative esophagitis, esophageal stricture, or Barrett's esophagus, APIs have a very clear edge of efficacy and should be considered first-line therapy.[31]

Only about 5% to 10% of patients with erosive esophagitis will fail to heal within 3 months on standard doses of APIs.[36]

Although in the majority of patients with moderate to severe peptic esophagitis the immediate problem can be controlled with short-term API therapy, current indications are that the minimum level of acid suppression needed to achieve healing is also the level needed for prevention of relapse.[31] Thus most such patients will need long-term maintenance therapy.

According to all available data, acid pump inhibition is effective for long-term control of moderate to severe esophagitis.[31] Lansoprazole and omeprazole has been found to be far more effective than both the placebo and the H_2-RA ranitidine in the maintenance treatment of GERD over a 12-month period.[37-39]

TABLE 7.4 — COMPARATIVE TRIALS OF LANSOPRAZOLE (30 MG DAILY) AND OMEPRAZOLE (20 MG DAILY) IN PATIENTS WITH ENDOSCOPICALLY CONFIRMED REFLUX ESOPHAGITIS

Reference	Study Design	Drug (no. of evaluable patients)	Healing Rate (% of Patients)			Relief of heart-burn at 2-4 wks
			2 wks	4 wks	8 wks	
Corallo et al*	db, mc, pg, r	L (76) O (69)	— —	86 84	88 88	L ≡ O
Hatlebakk et al	db, mc, pg, r	L (113) O (112)	— —	63 65	85 86.5	L > O†
Sekiguchi et al	Study design not specified	L (35) O (33)	76 63	97 76	— —	L > O

* Published in abstract form

† $p = 0.03$ between treatments at 4 weeks

db = double bind; mc = multicenter; pg = parallel group; r = randomized; ° indicates equivalent to comparator; > indicates superior to comparator.

Spencer CM, Faulds D. Lansoprazole: a reappraisal of its pharmacodynamic and pharmacokinetic properties, and its therapeutic efficacy in acid-related disorders. *Drugs*. 1994;48:418. Reprinted with permission.

REFERENCES

1. Dent J. Long-term aims of treatment of reflux disease, and the role of non-drug measures. *Digestion*. 1992;51 (suppl 1):30-34.

2. Garnett WR. Efficacy, safety and cost issues in managing patients with gastroesophageal reflux disease. *Am J Hosp Pharm*. 1993;50(suppl 1):S11-S18.

3. West JB. *Best and Taylor's Physiological Basis of Medical Practice*, 12th ed. Baltimore, Md: Williams & Wilkins; 1991:652-723.

4. Bullock J, Boyle J, Wang MB. *Physiology*, 2nd ed. Philadelphia, Pa: Harwal Publishing; 1990:310-317.

5. Feldman M. Gastric secretion. In: Sleisenger MH, Fordtran JS, ed. *Gastrointestinal Disease. Pathophysiology, Diagnosis, Management*. 3rd ed. Philadelphia, Pa: WB Saunders; 1983:541-558.

6. Higgs RH, Smyth RD, Castell DO. Gastric alkalinization:. Effect on lower-esophageal-sphincter pressure and serum gastrin. *N Engl J Med*. 1974;291:486-490.

7. Lipsy RJ, Fennerty B, Fagan TC. Clinical review of histamine$_2$-receptor antagonists. *Arch Intern Med*. 1990;150: 745-751.

8. Ippoliti A. Inflammatory and infectious esophageal disorders. In: Gitnick G, ed. *Principles and Practice of Gastroenterology and Hepatology*, 2nd ed. Norwalk, Conn: Appleton & Lange; 1994:37-49.

9. Sontag SJ. The medical management of reflux esophagitis. Role of antacids and acid inhibition. *Gastroenterol Clin North Am*. 1990;19:683-712.

10. Goodman and Gilman's.*The Pharmacologic Basis of Therapeutics*, 8th ed. New York, NY: Pergamon Press; 1990:899-904.

11. Morton LS, Fromkes JJ. Gastroesophageal reflux disease: diagnosis and medical therapy. *Geriatrics*. 1993;48:60-66.

12. Hixson LJ, Kelley CL, Jones WN, Tuohy CD. Current trends in the pharamcology for gastroesophageal reflux disease. *Arch Intern Med.* 1992;152:717-723.

13. Quigley EMM. Gastroesophageal reflux disease: the roles of motility in pathophysiology and therapy. *Am J Gastroenterol.* 1993;88:1649-1651.

14. Jensen SL, Jensen PF. Role of sucralfate in peptic disease. *Dig Dis Sci.* 1992;10:153-161.

15. McCarthy DM. Sucralfate. *N Engl J Med.* 1991;325: 1017-1025.

16. Ros E, Toledo-Pimentel V, Bordas JM, Grande L, Lacima G, Segu L. Healing of erosive esophagitis with sucralfate and cimetidine: influence of pretreatment lower esophageal sphincter pressure and serum pepsinogen I levels. *Am J Med.* 1991;92(suppl 2A):107S-113S.

17. Bremner CG, Marks IN, Segal I, Simjee A. Reflux esophagitis therapy: sucralfate versus ranitidine in a double-blind multicenter trial. *Am J Med.* 1991;91(suppl 2A): 119S-122S.

18. Roine R, Hernández-Muñoz R, Baraona E, Greenstein R, Leiber CS. Effect of omeprazole on gastric first-pass metabolism of ethanol. *Dig Dis Sci.* 1992;37:891-896.

19. Ramirez B, Richter JE. Review article: promotility drugs in the treatment of gastro-oesophageal reflux disease. *Aliment Pharmacol Ther.* 1993;7:5-20.

20. Galmiche JP, Brandstätter G, Evreux M, et al. Combined therapy with cisapride and cimetidine in severe reflux oesophagitis: a double-blind controlled trial. *Gut.* 1988; 29:675-681.

21. Weinbeck M, The Ranpride Study Group. Does cisapride added to H_2-receptor-blocking treatment improve healing rates in patients with esophagitis? *Digestion.* 1986;34: 144A. Abstract.

22. Maton PN. Omeprazole. *N Engl J Med.* 1991;324:965-975.

23. Smolka A, Helender HF, Sachs G. Monoclonal antibodies against gastric H^+/K^+-ATPase. *Gastrointest Liver Physiol.* 1983;245:G589-G596.

24. Mohamed AH, Hunt RH. The rationale of acid suppression in the treatment of acid-related disease. *Aliment Pharmacol Ther.* 1994;8(suppl 1):3-10.

25. Karnes WE Jr, Walsh JH. The gastrin hypothesis. Implications for antisecretory drug selection. *J Clin Gastroenterol.* 1990;12(suppl 2):S7-S12.

26. McTavish D, Buckley MM, Heel RC. Omeprazole. An updated review of its pharmacology and therapeutic use in acid-related disorders. *Drugs.* 1991;42:138-170.

27. *Physicians' Desk Reference®*, 51st ed. Montvale, NJ: Medical Economics Data Production Company; 1997: 2746-2748.

28. Spencer CM, Faulds D. Lansoprazole. A reappraisal of its pharmacodynamic and pharmacokinetic properties, and its therapeutic efficacy in acid-related disorders. *Drugs.* 1994;48:404-430.

29. *Physicians' Desk Reference®*, 51st ed. Montvale, NJ: Medical Economics Data Production Company; 1997: 516-519.

30. Eisen SA, Miller DK, Woodward RS, Spitznagel E, Przybeck TR. The effect of prescribed daily dose frequency on patient medication compliance. *Arch Intern Med.* 1990;150:1881-1884.

31. Arens MJ, Dent J. Acid pump blockers: what are their current therapeutic roles? *Baillieres Clin Gastroenterol.* 1993;7:95-128.

32. Robinson M, Campbell DR, Sontag S, Sabesin SM. Treatment of erosive reflux esophagitis resistant to H_2-receptor antagonist therapy. Lansoprazole, a new proton pump inhibitor. *Dig Dis Sci.* 1995;40:590-597.

33. Feldman M, Harford WV, Fisher RS, et al. Treatment of reflux esophagitis resistant to H_2-receptor antagonists with lansoprazole, a new H^+/K^+-ATPase inhibitor: a controlled, double-blind study. Lansoprazole Study Group. *Am J Gastroenterol.* 1993;88:1212-1217.

34. Castell DO, Richter JE, Robinson M, Sontag SJ, Haber MM. Efficacy and safety of lansoprazole in the treatment of erosive reflux esophagitis. The Lansoprazole Group. *Am J Gastroenterol.* 1996;91:1749-1757.

35. Mee AS, Rowley JL, the Lansoprazole Clinical Research Group. Rapid symptom relief in reflux oesophagitis: a comparison of lansoprazole and omeprazole. *Ailment Pharmacol Ther.* 1996;10:757-763.

36. Bardhan KD. Is there any acid peptic disease that is refractory to proton pump inhibitors? *Aliment Pharmacol Ther.* 1993;7(suppl 1):13-31.

37. Robinson M, Lanza F, the Lansoprazole Study Group. Lansoprazole for one year prevents recurrence of erosive reflux esophagitis. *Gastroenterology.* 1994;106:A166. Abstract.

38. Swarbrick ET, Gough AL, Christian J, et al. Prevention of recurrence of oesophageal stricture. A comparative study of lansoprazole and high dose ranitidine. *Gastroenterology.* 1994;106:A189. Abstract.

39. Lundell L. Prevention of relapse of reflux oesophagitis after endoscopic healing: the efficiency and safety of omeprazole compared to ranitidine. *Digestion.* 1990;47 (suppl 1):72-75.

8 Surgical Management

The development of more effective histamine$_2$-receptor antagonist (H_2-RA) dosing schedules plus the introduction of the acid pump inhibitors (APIs), which completely resolve symptoms and heal esophagitis in the majority of patients with severe gastroesophageal reflux disease (GERD), might seem to make antireflux surgery obsolete.[1] Not so. Rather, the greatly improved medical interventions have helped identify patients most likely to benefit from surgical intervention.

Antireflux surgery should be reserved for patients with complicated GERD who will require lifetime medical therapy.[1] Although there can be no hard-and-fast rules, reasonable indications for surgery include:[1]

- Refractory reflux disease with intolerable symptoms or esophagitis that has proved difficult to treat
- Recurrent esophageal strictures
- Esophagotracheal aspiration resulting in recurrent pneumonia, asthma, or laryngitis
- Bleeding from Barrett's ulcers or as a result of a hiatal hernia causing linear gastric erosions.

Barrett's esophagus is not by itself an indication for surgery since columnar epithelium does not predictably regress with successful control of acid reflux.[1] Thus, even after successful surgery, patients continue to require surveillance for carcinoma.

Careful preoperative evaluation of esophageal function is crucial to identifying surgical candidates. Diagnostic procedures should include:[1]

- Endoscopy
- Manometric assessment of the functional motor capacity of the esophageal body
- Long-term (24-hour) esophageal pH monitoring during optimal medical treatment.

If 24-hour esophageal pH monitoring is normal in a patient with unequivocal endoscopic esophagitis, the possibilities of alkaline, drug-induced, or retention esophagitis should be considered.[2,3] Older patients with recent-onset esophagitis and esophageal stricture should raise particular suspicions of drug-induced disease.

Several factors will influence whether and what kind of surgery is required:[3]

- Functional status of the esophageal body
- Esophageal length
- Presence of hypersecretion
- Degree of delayed gastric emptying, if present
- Age and general condition (surgical risk).

■ Esophageal Body Motility

Patients with normal peristaltic function do well with the most common antireflux procedure, a 360-degree Nissen fundoplication.[3] When peristalsis is absent, severely disordered, or of low magnitude, however, the Belsey two-thirds partial fundoplication may be the operation of choice. Thus, the propulsive force of the esophageal body should be evaluated manometrically to determine its ability to propel a bolus of food through a newly constructed valve.[3]

■ Esophageal Length

A short esophagus, often associated with stricture, Barrett's esophagus, or a large hiatal hernia, can compromise the surgeon's ability to achieve an adequate repair without tension, leading to its possible breakdown or thoracic displacement.[3] In patients with a hiatal hernia, shortening is identified on barium esophagoscopy or on endoscopy. On x-ray, the hernia will not reduce with the patient in the upright position, or, on direct visualization, the measurement between the diaphragmatic crura and the gastroesophageal junction (GEJ) is more than 5 cm. A short esophagus may require lengthening, usually with a Colles gastroplasty, but only after motility evaluation of the esophageal body. In the presence of no motility, more than 70% ineffective contractions, or several failed procedures, esophageal resection should be considered.

■ Hypersecretion

Approximately 30% of patients with pathologic esophageal reflux on pH monitoring will have hypersecretion on gastric analysis.[3] Among these patients who undergo antireflux surgery, 2% to 3% will develop a gastric or duodenal ulcer. Therefore, in a patient with either concurrent or a history of ulcer disease, the surgical procedure may be modified by the addition of vagotomy.

■ Delayed Gastric Emptying

Delayed gastric emptying is found in approximately 40% of patients with GERD and can contribute to symptoms after surgery.[3] As a rule, however, mild delays are corrected by the antireflux procedure.[4]

■ Surgical Procedures

Unlike surgery to remove a diseased organ, which will be destroyed with its removal, antireflux surgery is designed to improve the function of an intact organ.[3] Its goal is to provide complete and permanent relief of all symptoms and complications of gastroesophageal reflux secondary to an incompetent lower esophageal stricture (LES).

The most common antireflux operation worldwide is the Nissen (360-degree) fundoplication.[3] Other procedures include two partial fundoplications, the Belsey (270-degree) and the Toupet (180-degree), and the Hill posterior gastropexy.[1] Each involves reduction of a hiatal hernia, if present, as well as construction of a valve mechanism. Each of the procedures provides good to excellent relief of reflux symptoms in 84% to 89% of patients (Table 8.1).[3] Furthermore, each has its own strengths and weaknesses, and may be applicable in specific situations (Table 8.2).

Recent advances in laparoscopic instrumentation and technique now allow surgical fundoplication with video control.[5] Indications for the laparoscopic approach are the same as those for open surgery. Neither obesity nor previous surgery are absolute contraindications, although, as in open surgery, both make the procedure more demanding.

Antireflux procedures, open or laparoscopic, should be performed only by skilled personnel with particular interest and experience in the management of GERD and in centers with all essential diagnostic, therapeutic, and surgical facilities.[1]

TABLE 8.1 — RESULTS OF PRIMARY SURGICAL ANTIREFLUX REPAIRS FOR GERD

Repair	Source	No. of Patients	Follow-up Period	Good Results (%)	Reflux Recurrence (%)	Dysphagia (%)	Gas Bloat (%)	Mortality (%)
Belsey	Skinner	632	1-5 yrs	85	7.0	—	—	1.2
Mark IV	Orringer	892	3-15 yrs	84	11.0	—	—	1.0
Hill posterior gastropexy	Hill 1967, 1983	149	—	—	4.8	2	—	
	No intraoperative motility	541	—	—	4.8	—	—	0
	Intraoperative motility	191	—	—	1.5	—	—	—
	No intraoperative motility	72	92.6 mos	65	4.1	0	—	0
	Intraoperative	83	47 mos	89	0	0	—	0
	Maher 1978	65	—	82	9	—	—	4.6
Nissen	Five reports	1141	1-12 yrs	87	7	8 (4/48)	8 (97/1115)	1.0

DeMeester TR, Stein HJ. Surgical treatment of gastroesophageal reflux disease. In: Castell DO, ed. *The Esophagus*. Boston, Mass: Little, Brown & Company; 1992:615. Reprinted with permission.

8

TABLE 8.2 — COMPARISON OF CURRENT ANTIREFLUX PROCEDURES

Operation	Concept of Function	Ease of Construction	Effectiveness of Valve	Outflow Resistance	Toleration of Tension	Best Use
Hill posterior gastropexy	Complex	Difficult	Dependent on intraoperative manometrics	Dependent on degree of imbrication of cardia	Good	Previous gastric resection
Belsey partial fundoplication	Simple	Most difficult	Effective; patient usually able to belch	Lowest	Poor	Poor esophageal pump
Nissen fundoplication	Simple	Average	Most effective; patient unable to belch	Highest; long and tight wrap can cause permanent dysphagia	Fair	Standard antireflux procedure
Collis Belsey (Pearson procedure)	Simple	Difficult	Effective; patient unable to belch	Low	Best	Poor esophageal pump and short esophagus

DeMeester TR, Stein HJ. Surgical treatment of gastroesophageal reflux disease. In: Castell DO, ed. *The Esophagus*. Boston, Mass: Little, Brown; 1992;614. Reprinted with permission.

REFERENCES

1. Richter JE. Surgery for reflux disease—reflections of a gastroenterologist. *N Engl J Med.* 1992;326:825-827. Editorial.

2. Bonavina L, DeMeester TR, McChesney L, Schwizer W, Albertucci M, Bailey RT. Drug-induced esophageal strictures. *Ann Surg*. 1987;206:173-183.

3. Peters JH, DeMeester TR. Gastroesophageal reflux. *Surg Clin North Am*. 1993;73:1119-1144.

4. Hinder RA, Stein HJ, Bremner CG, DeMeester TR. Relationship of a satisfactory outcome to normalization of delayed gastric emptying after Nissen fundoplication. *Ann Surg*. 1989;210:458-465.

5. Salky B. Who is a candidate for laparoscopic fundoplication? Will it become the procedure of choice? Syllabus. NY Soc Gastrointest Endoc Postgrad Course. November 10-11, 1994:1.

INDEX

Note: Page numbers in *italics* indicate figures; page numbers followed by t indicate tables.